The Run Walk Run® I.

JEFF GALLOWAY

THE **RUN WALK RUN**®
METHOD

THIRD EDITION

Meyer & Meyer Sport

British Library of Cataloguing in Publication Data
A catalogue record for this book is available from the British Library

The Run Walk Run® Method
Maidenhead: Meyer & Meyer Sport (UK) Ltd., 2025
ISBN 978-1-78255-271-0

© 2013, 2016, 2025 by Meyer & Meyer Sport (UK) Ltd.
Third edition 2025.

Aachen, Auckland, Beirut, Cairo, Cape Town, Dubai, Hägendorf, Hong Kong,
Indianapolis, Manila, New Delhi, Singapore, Sydney, Tehran, Vienna

Member of the World Sport Publishers' Association (WSPA) www.w-s-p-a.org

Printed by Versa Press, East Peoria, IL
Printed in the United States of America
ISBN 978-1-78255-271-0
E-Mail: info@m-m-sports.com
www.thesportspublisher.com

Contents

Introduction		7
Chapter 1	Run Walk Run Brings Us Back to Our Roots	12
Chapter 2	The Galloway Run Walk Run (RWR) Method	14
Chapter 3	Are You Really a Runner If You Walk?	18
Chapter 4	Principles Behind Run Walk Run	24
Chapter 5	The Mental Benefits of Run Walk Run	28
Chapter 6	How Can the Run Walk Run Method Eliminate Injury?	32
Chapter 7	The Magic Mile Time Trial Guides the Run Walk Run Strategy	36
Chapter 8	Setting Up the Right Run Walk Run Strategy	46
Chapter 9	How to Keep Track of the Walk Breaks	54
Chapter 10	GET OFF THE COUCH! Run Walk Run for Beginners	58
Chapter 11	Running Form—Walk Breaks Help You Adapt to Efficient Movement	66
Chapter 12	Walking Form	70
Chapter 13	Drills to Transition From Running to Walking and Back Again	74
Chapter 14	Solving Problems by Adjusting Run Walk Run Strategies	80
Chapter 15	Running Faster With Run Walk Run	108
Chapter 16	Race Rehearsal	112
Chapter 17	Making Adjustments Using Run Walk Run	116
Chapter 18	Motivation Strategies Using Run Walk Run	120
Chapter 19	Run Walk Run Issues and Problems	128
Chapter 20	Variations to the Traditional Running and Walking Intervals	
	by Dr. Stanley Zaslau	134
Chapter 21	Products That Enhance Running	138
Chapter 22	Testimonials	162
Index		188

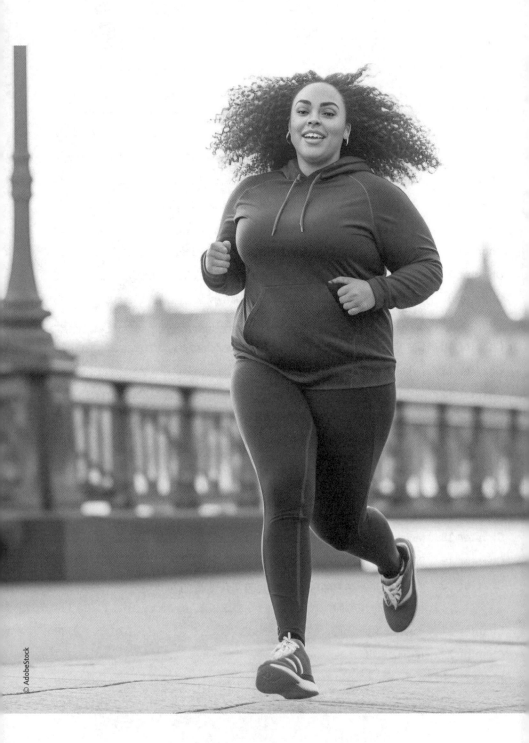

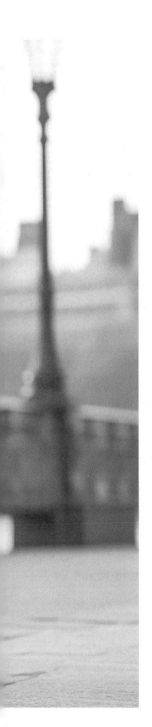

Introduction

All the joys of running—without the pain!

Running turns on brain circuits for a better attitude, more vitality, and personal empowerment better than other activities studied. Millions start and re-start their running career because they know they will feel better, think better, and enjoy life better if they run regularly but break down in pain or exhaustion because they run non-stop.

My Run Walk Run (RWR) method can take away the pain and bring the joy of running to almost everyone. Veteran runners are running faster and avoiding injuries. Millions of new runners are discovering that strategic walk breaks leave them feeling good during and after a run, able to enjoy family, career and social activities with the mindset of an athlete.

As you might imagine, these converts to the method are telling their friends, and showing them how to experience these life-changing enhancements at any age. As each new Run Walk Runner infects at least 10 others to try the method, a new running boom is spreading across the globe.

Shoe and clothing manufacturers are not making enough of the popular running products. Races are expanding and popular ones are filling up sooner than ever. So many of these new runners were quite comfortable, sedentary citizens before deciding to take on a series of rigorous physical challenges. Why did they do this?

Feedback from hundreds of thousands of runners over the past 40 years has a consistent theme. Even a confirmed couch sitter can receive a sense of empowerment and joy not experienced in other activities. Once these enhancements are experienced, who wants to go back to the old life?

When talking to groups of new runners, most tell me that they didn't even consider trying it until they heard about Run Walk Run. Many of them tried to run non-stop for short distances and had to stop within a city block or less due to pain, excess breathing, or failure of the running muscles. As soon as they used the right Run Walk Run strategy, a whole new world opened up.

Almost everyone wants to have control over their destiny. Run Walk Run allows each of us to be the captain of our running ship, adjusting the running, the walking, and the pace, so that one can get the workout desired...without the negatives of overexertion.

Ten years ago, in major races, about ten percent of the runners were taking walk breaks. Observers today estimate that about 40-50% are using the Run Walk Run method in some form—and the percentage is growing every year. According to thousands of reports every year, the Galloway RWR method is the only reason that many novice runners thought that they could even try to run. Within a year or two they are finishing marathons and half marathons. You know who they are—the ones who are passing others during the last few miles of the race.

There are few things in life more exhilarating than passing people at the end of a race.

Because each runner can control the amount of running and the amount of walking, each can be successful every day. Without the pressure of having to run for any specific distance, every running moment can be enjoyed, as friends can talk and laugh during a workout.

Surprisingly, veterans are running faster with the right placement of walk breaks. Not only are energy reserves and muscle resources conserved. Adaptations are made and fatigue is erased during the race so that Run Walk Runners are strong to the end, passing others. This activates the will to do one's best which non-stop runners tend to lose by the end of a hard race or workout.

There are many tools in this book that give the individual control over his or her destiny. The most powerful effect of the Run Walk Run strategy is the activation of the most effective tool we have: the conscious brain. As we set up the right ratio of running to walking each day, we turn on circuits in the executive brain that infuse energy, improve attitude, gear up physical systems, trigger positive hormones, and keep the components in synch and communicating with one another.

The regular use of this conscious brain gives us control over our experience. As we fine-tune our pace with the right Run Walk Run strategy we develop a sense of belief in the process of becoming better. Formerly confirmed sedentary citizens find themselves going out the door on an oppressively cold day because of the joy delivered by each run. Studies show that as one gets into running, dietary choices tend to become more healthy, work productivity increases, and runners look for and find other ways of improving the quality of their life.

The daily empowerment from balancing running and walking is reinforcing but the greatest reward is the positive activation of the spirit. That mysterious positive will to go on is what makes us uniquely human. Of all of the activities that offer spiritual enhancement, running is one of the most comprehensive: bringing together body mind and spirit as a powerful team.

Every year I meet and talk to runners ages 4 to 84 and have met with runners in all continents except Antarctica. We share the same positive enhancements. The best part is that most can run for the rest of their lives....with the right Run Walk Run adjustments.

Run Walk Run: The Beginning

In 1974 I was asked to teach a class in beginning running. I had opened my specialty running store, Phidippides, and wanted to help average citizens enjoy the benefits of running. Honestly, I also wanted to increase the number of potential customers.

During the first class I discovered that none of my students had been running for at least five years. About one-third had never done any regularly scheduled exercise. During the first lap around the track I realized that walk breaks would be crucial if I wanted each class member to finish either a 5K or 10K without injury or exhaustion.

Three pace groups naturally emerged. The beginners called themselves basket case physical specimens. At the other end of the conditioning spectrum was a group of young guys who had been regularly engaged in other sports and were in good shape. There was also a middle group. As I ran with each group on each workout I focused on breathing rate. The huff-and-puff rule emerged: when you hear huffing and puffing increase, take more frequent walk breaks and slow the pace.

Throughout the first class I adjusted the Run Walk Run amounts so that each person felt successful in completing the distance—which gradually increased during one run each week. Most admitted that they started to look forward to each run because of the improved attitude during and afterward.

At the end of the 10-week term was the exam: either a 5K or 10K. Each student—even the self-titled basket cases—finished one or the other. When I polled each at the end, I received my best reward: none of them had been injured.

I had never been with a group of 20 or more runners for more than two months without some injuries. When my novices had started to feel aches I increased the frequency of walk breaks and their bodies adapted.

During the next two years I experimented with various ratios of walk breaks as I worked with beginning runners who ran in groups from my store, and in individual consultations. In 1976 Galloway training programs began. I continued to find that walk breaks could almost eliminate injury.

Many of the veteran marathoners refused to take walk breaks at first. As the former beginners moved into longer distance events such as marathons, they continued to adjust walk breaks and started to record faster times than the veterans. This led to the use of walk breaks in all of the pace groups.

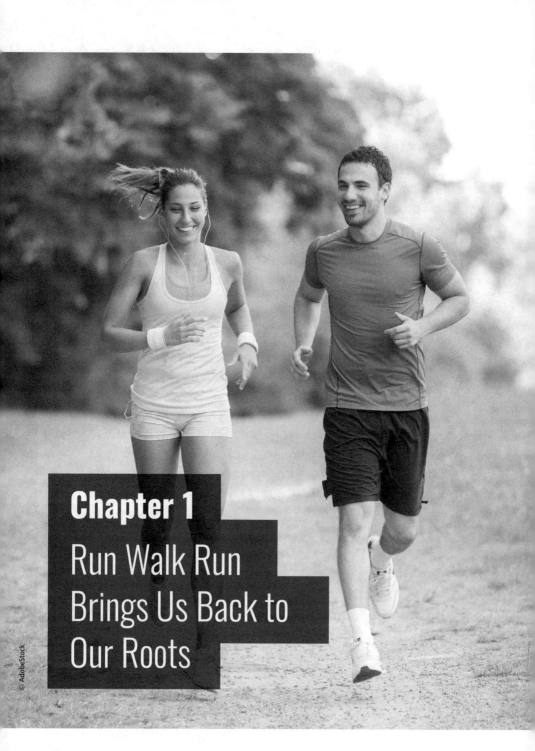

© AdobeStock

Chapter 1

Run Walk Run
Brings Us Back to
Our Roots

Anthropologists who study ancient man have told me they don't believe humans were originally suited for continuous long-distance running. Over the millions of years that our ancestors moved from four feet to two feet for transportation, they walked long distances every day and developed extremely efficient movement patterns.

Indeed, survival was enhanced by the ability to keep moving every day and to gather limited supplies of food—while spending minimum amounts of energy. These experts believe that running was used in relatively short bursts to get away from predators, jump over obstacles and later in the evolutionary cycle, to pick up the pace when tracking animals.

Increased energy consumption. We can adapt to continuous running, but at the cost of dramatically faster expenditure of limited energy supplies and muscle resources. We must lift our body weight off the ground with each running step—and absorb the shock of landing. Running continuously will result in an energy crisis which forces thousands of non-stop marathoners each year to mostly walk during the last 4-6 miles of their marathon.

Reduced orthopedic stress. Continuous running greatly increases the aggravation on the orthopedic system, compared with the very minor irritations of walking. The walk motion uses momentum very efficiently through biomechanics that have been adapted, fine-tuned, and upgraded for millions of years. Everyone has a few weak links in the orthopedic system that become targets during non-stop running and break down sooner due to range of motion, genetics, prior injury, etc.

Simply stated, we can train ourselves to run continuously for increasingly longer distance. But the accumulation of stress on weak links will eventually reach a level where the joint, muscle, tendon, etc. will fail. This often requires weeks or months of repair.

Run Walk Run is a strategy to eliminate break down. Inserting the walks before the weak link is damaged allows stress to be managed, repaired, and adapted, while other areas are recruited to get the job done. It's possible to stay injury free while continuing to increase distance with the early and regular insertion of walk breaks. This ancient method allows us to be in charge of our running future.

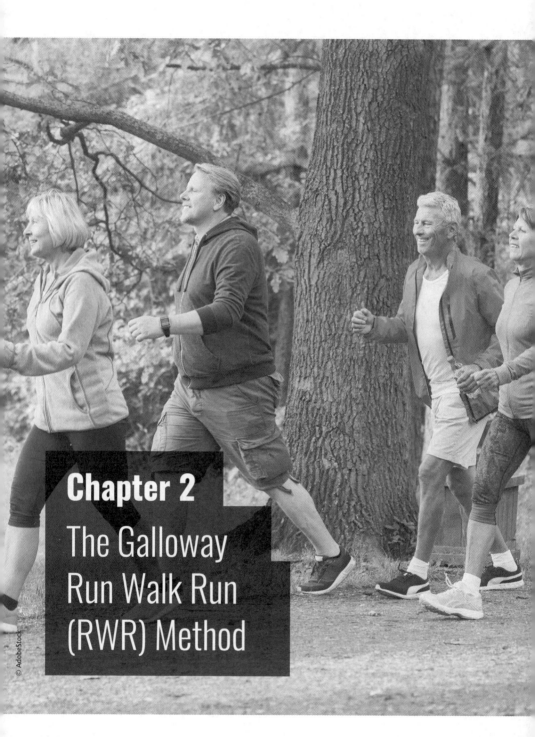

Chapter 2

The Galloway Run Walk Run (RWR) Method

© AdobeStock

- A smart way to run—by giving you cognitive control over each workout
- Allows you to carry on all of your life activities—even after long runs
- Motivates beginners to get off the couch and run
- Bestows running joy to non-stop runners who had given up due to injury or burnout
- Helps improve finish times in races
- Gives all runners control over fatigue
- Delivers all of the running enhancements without exhaustion or pain
- Allows YOU to make the rules for your run each day
- Strategic rest interval—walk before you get tired
- A short and gentle walking stride
- No need to eliminate the walk breaks

Strategic rest interval—walk before you get tired

Most of us, even when untrained, can walk for several miles before fatigue sets in, because we're genetically designed to walk efficiently for hours. Running is more work, because you have to lift your body off the ground and then absorb the shock of the landing, over and over.

The continuous use of the running muscles will produce more fatigue, aches, and pains than maintaining the same pace while taking walk breaks. If you walk before your running muscles start to get tired, you allow the muscle to recover instantly—increasing your capacity for exercise while reducing the chance of next-day soreness.

The method part involves having a strategy. By using a ratio of running and walking that is right for you on each day, you can manage your fatigue. The result? You're the one who is strong to the finish, doing what you need or want to do after long runs. You never have to be exhausted after a long run again.

The RWR method is very simple—you run for a short segment and then take a walk break, and keep repeating this pattern.

Walk Breaks...

- Increase speed an average of 7 minutes faster in a 13.1-mile race when non-stop runners shift to the correct Run Walk Run ratio—and more than 13 minutes faster in the marathon (average improvement based upon statistical surveys)
- Give you control over the way you feel during and afterward
- Erase fatigue
- Push back your wall of exhaustion or soreness
- Allow for endorphins to collect during each walk break—you feel good!
- Break up the distance into manageable units (e.g., "Just 30 seconds until a walk break!")
- Speed recovery
- Reduce the chance of aches, pains, and injury
- Allow you to feel good afterward—carrying on the rest of your day without debilitating fatigue
- Give you all of the endurance and empowerment of the distance of each workout—without the pain
- Allow older runners or heavier runners to recover quickly, and feel as good or better as the younger (slimmer) days
- Activate the frontal lobe, maintaining your control over attitude and motivation

A short and gentle walking stride

It's better to walk slowly, with a short stride. There has been some irritation of the shins, when runners or walkers maintain a stride that is too long. Relax and enjoy the walk.

No need to eliminate the walk breaks

Some beginners assume that they must work toward the day when they don't have to take any walk breaks at all. This is up to the individual, but it is not recommended. Remember that you choose the Run Walk Run strategy for that day. There is no rule that requires you to hold to any configuration on a given day. As you adjust the running and the walking to how you feel, you gain control over your fatigue.

I've run for over 50 years, and I enjoy running more than ever because of walk breaks. Each run I take energizes my day. I would not be able to run almost every day if I didn't insert the walk breaks early and often.

Run Walk Run allows YOU to make the rules for your run, each day.

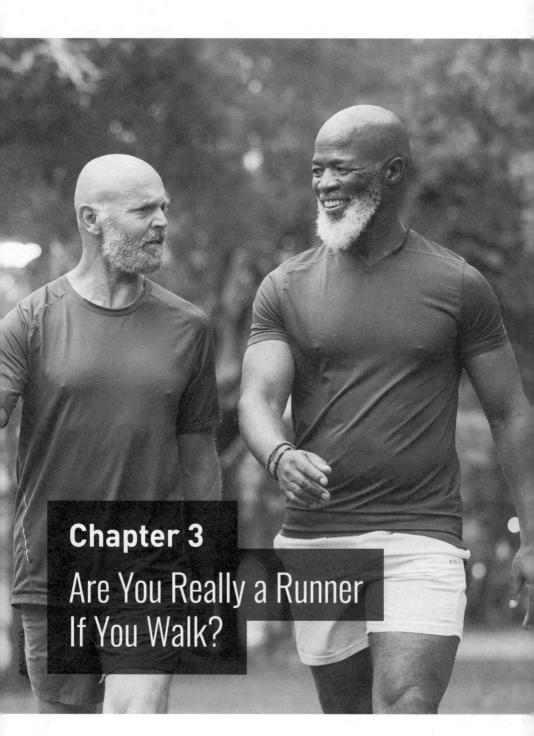

Chapter 3

Are You Really a Runner
If You Walk?

Almost every day a new runner reports to me that an experienced runner said something like this: "If you take walk breaks, you're not a runner."

When someone says this to me my comeback is the following:

"I've been on the U.S. Olympic team and have run for more than 50 years, and I didn't know that there was a running rule book that excludes walking. Could you show me in the rulebook ?"

There is no list of rules. The most wonderful aspect about running, compared to other sports, is that each of us determines where, when, how far, and how fast to run. We are the captains of our running ships and have complete control over how we do it each day.

But in almost every aspect of our lives there are a few people who believe that their way of doing things is the only way. They have no right to tell anyone how he or she should run, but they were around when I took my first running steps in 1958, telling me that I wasn't running correctly unless I did it *their* way. When I made training changes that allowed me to qualify for the U.S. Olympic team, some of them told me I wasn't running enough while others said I was running too much. Unlike most runners who are supportive and want to help other runners, this tiny percentage of narcissists often picks on beginners because they are impressionable. Unfortunately I meet a number of former beginners who stopped running because of such negative coaching.

If we ran as the first marathoners ran, we should all be taking walk breaks. Marathon competition began in 1896, in the first edition of the modern Olympic Games. A few years ago, while wandering through a museum in Athens, Greece, I noticed a newspaper column on display with a picture of the winner of this first marathon race. Our Greek guide, Maria, translated the account of a reporter who followed the runners from start to finish. The quote that I will always remember is: *"Every one of the athletes walked significantly in this race."*

I will never try to drag anyone kicking and screaming into Run Walk Run. Each runner can choose to run or walk as much or as little as they wish. The benefits are numerous, but some runners believe that running means no walking at all in a race or workout. There are only a handful of runners who do this on all of their runs. A runner has the right to insist that non-stop running is the only way to run for himself or herself—but no right to impose this on anyone else.

You don't even have to answer the usually negative remarks made by these runners. You have a proven method that can get you to finish any run with strength, and never be out of commission for friends and family.

You are the captain of your running—and walking—ship.

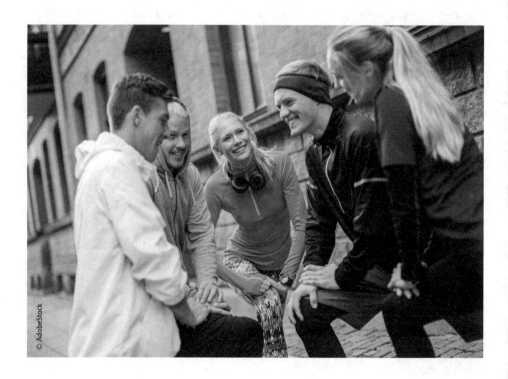

© AdobeStock

How to reprogram the subconscious reflex brain to use Run Walk Run.

Most children have been instructed while in physical education class or on a sports team to never walk. A common coaching statement that is embedded in the subconscious reflex brain is that walking is failure. There are reasons why coaches will instruct their students to keep running during short events, but it is neither necessary nor productive to follow this advice for the rest of our lives.

It's a fact that this childhood programming is very powerful and hardwired as a subconscious reflex behavior pattern. When we start to take a walk break, even 20 years after we finished our last cross country race or PE class, stress builds up in the reflex brain and anxiety hormones are produced. This subconscious brain may also trigger your memory to remind you what your coach said (or at least a fuzzy remembrance).

But there's hope. We can reprogram the reflex brain to accept the taking of walk breaks as normal by using a cognitive strategy. This shifts control away from the subconscious and into the executive center that does the retraining. Here's how.

1. Use the Magic Mile to determine a realistic goal pace and a conservative long run pace.

2. Set your Run Walk Run ratio based upon the pace per mile of both the goal pace and the long run pace using the Galloway Run Walk Run strategy in chapter 7.

3. Load yourself up with all the positive Run Walk Run mantras and key phrases. Memorize these or write them down so that you can talk back to the reflex brain's negative messages:

   • Walk breaks make me strong—to the end.

- Walk breaks allow me to do what I want to the rest of the day.

- Walk breaks speed my recovery.

- Walk breaks help me run faster.

- Walk breaks let me control fatigue.

- Walk breaks break up the distance into doable segments.

- Walk breaks give me control over my running enjoyment.

4. Use the Galloway Run-Walk-Run app or program your watch for segments. The app is available from all app stores and gets you into a rhythmic pattern of RWR. This is a great way to reprogram the reflex brain.

5. At the end of each run, make a conscious statement about how the Run Walk Run method is superior to your old way—"I have a tool to enjoy running for life."

You determine how much you run and how much you walk.

One of the wonderful aspects of running is that there is no definition of a runner that you must live up to. There are also no rules that you must follow as you do your daily run. You are the captain of your running ship and it is you who determines how far, how fast, and how much you will run, walk, etc. While you will hear many opinions on this, running has always been a freestyle type of activity in which *each individual is empowered to mix and match the many variables* and come out with the running experience that he or she chooses. Walk breaks can keep the first-time runner away from injury and burnout, and can help veterans to improve time.

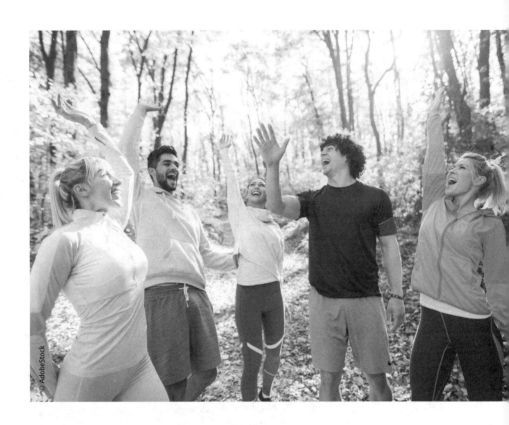

© AdobeStock

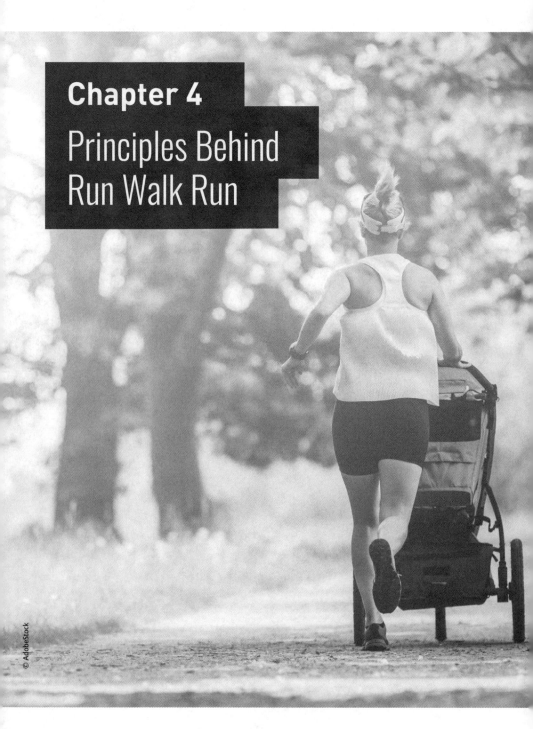

Chapter 4
Principles Behind Run Walk Run

© AdobeStock

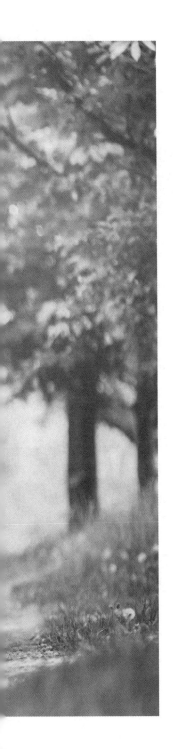

The next chapter will highlight the mental benefits of the method. I believe that the most empowering part of Run Walk Run is that it is a cognitive strategy—giving you control over your exercise, attitude, fatigue, and energy.

Our human organism is designed to improve and repair itself when a gentle stress is followed by a recovery period. Running continuously will cause a stress buildup that can be eliminated when walk breaks are taken early and often. During each walk, the body's systems can adapt, the orthopedic units can rebuild and restore themselves. Here are some of the principles behind this process.

- **Continuous use of a muscle results in quicker fatigue.** During a walk break the muscle can adapt, recover, erase fatigue, and rebound to perform better and longer.

- **The longer the run segment, the more fatigue.** Many runners run faster by reducing the run segment and walking more frequently.

- **Run Walk Run is a form of interval training.** The human organism can handle a gentle increase in stress if there is a recovery interval regularly inserted. Knowledgeable coaches have used this interval training concept for over a hundred years to prepare athletes for increased distance and speed.

- **Conservation of resources.** Running continuously uses up energy resources and muscle performance more quickly. When walk breaks are inserted early and often enough, there is more fuel in the tank later in the run. In addition, muscles are revived during each walk break. This means little or no slowdown at the end.

- **Elimination of cramping.** After analyzing the reports from thousands who have cramped during training runs and races, I've found that the leading cause is non-stop running. The right Run Walk Run strategy, from the beginning, has eliminated cramping for most who have suffered from this painful experience.

- **Quicker recovery.** Walk breaks allow for muscles to recover faster from any workout. The earlier and the more frequently walk breaks are inserted, the quicker the recovery and the sooner one can resume the desired type of running. Time goal runners can do the strenuous speed sessions needed to improve. Fitness runners can resume regular activity, and enjoy activities with friends and family even after extremely long runs. Frequent walk breaks allow even first-year runners to enjoy the satisfaction of finishing half marathons, and even marathons, every month.

- **Less stress on the weak links.** Most runners experience downtime due the irritation of a few sites in a few body parts. Without using Run Walk Run, these aches, pains, and injuries occur over and over again, due to individual range of motion, genetics, etc. Running continuously will continue to build up the stress and damage, often resulting in an injury. Each walk break can release the stress buildup, allow the tissue to adapt, or shift workload to other areas. I've heard from hundreds of runners that had been diagnosed with serious orthopedic problems and assumed they would have to stop running. A liberal insertion of walking, from the beginning of all runs, has brought these folks back into running—often allowing for running longer distances again.

- **Enjoy endorphins during the run.** Endorphins help to manage pain from running and can deliver a side effect of improving attitude and injecting relaxation, making one feel better than before. The body organism stimulates endorphin release when one starts running. When running continuously, the endorphins tend to be needed to kill the pains and aggravation of running. Most runners experience the endorphin afterglow of a run, but Run Walk Runners can get the attitude boost during many of the walk breaks. Because a gentle walk doesn't generate continuing damage, there is no new pain produced. The endorphins can then inject their good attitude hormones into receptor sites in billions of cells throughout the body.

- **Reduce core body temperature increase.** Running is a lot more work than gentle walking, and produces a significant increase in the core body temperature on a hot day. Running on a day in which the temperature is 60°F (14°C) or higher will result in heat buildup, more sweating and dehydration, and more work for the body to keep you from overheating. Running continuously can keep building heat stress on the body, resulting in heat disease, slower times in races, longer recovery, and loss of desire to run. The early and frequent insertion of walk breaks has significantly reduced temperature increase in my clients who have had heat problems previously, allowing them to adapt to running in warm weather.

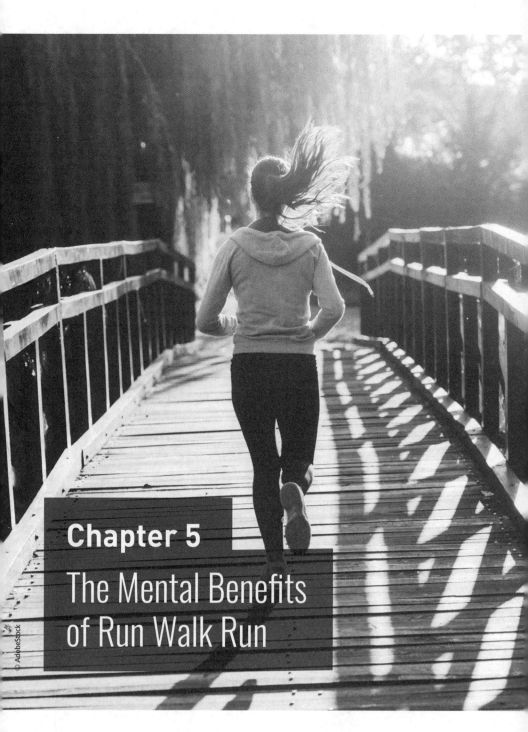

© AdobeStock

Chapter 5

The Mental Benefits
of Run Walk Run

While the physical benefits of the Run Walk Run method are amazing, the mental enhancements could be more significant. The motivation to run, or to improve, is influenced significantly by the various components of the brain. Stress in life and the stress of running can stimulate our subconscious brain to secrete negative attitude hormones.

But when we focus on the RWR method, this cognitive strategy shifts mental control to the conscious brain (the human brain—executive decision center) that can override the subconscious. By using a proven Run Walk Run strategy and believing in it, you can stop the production of negative hormones and stimulate positive hormones as you move forward. Just having a plan will reduce the sensation of stress and give one more control over attitude.

- You are the captain of your running ship. Having a strategy allows one to gain control over fatigue, aches and pains, breathing rate—over the run itself. Being in command reduces stress and is empowering by itself.

- Running helps us think better. Pre-test/post-test studies show that runners solve problems quicker and better after a run. Non-stop running tends to produce such a high level of stress, fatigue, and pain that mental focus shifts to the misery index. Frequent walk breaks release the physical stress, allowing the brain to be free to focus on other areas, and to create, think, and solve.

- Better mental energy. During a run, mental circuits are turned on that result in increased activity of logical and creative patterns in the frontal lobe. Early and frequent walk breaks allow the brain to shift gears and become energized. This increased level of activity can last for hours. I hear from countless runners every year who tell me the insertion of the right walk breaks made the difference.

Why do some runners have trouble taking walk breaks?

Research shows that the lessons learned in the early school years are powerfully embedded in the subconscious brain. While it is natural to feel anxious and then receive negative hormones when we depart from these hard-wired patterns, conscious actions can retrain this ancient brain. The cognitive focus on specific run segments and set amount of walks can hardwire new patterns into the reflex brain.

This gives you control over your attitude as you feel the positive results from using strategic walk breaks. Through the use of mantras and systematic actions, you empower the conscious brain to take control. This frontal lobe component can override the subconscious brain and retrain it to accept and embrace the Run Walk Run® method.

• Running can help you set up cognitive strategies for other areas in life. During the run, circuits are turned on in the conscious executive brain to solve running problems, watch for road hazards, increase heart rate, etc. This increased mental activity is often applied to problems at work, at home, hobbies, etc. Almost every day a runner will tell me that he or she had been struggling with a work issue for days or weeks and it was during a run that the solution was revealed. Walk breaks allow the mind to relax, shift gears, and be ready to solve problems.

• As you focus on each segment, you empower the conscious brain. Run Walk Run® is a cognitive strategy that can shift control to the conscious, executive brain. In the process, you can deny the subconscious brain its chance to secrete negative attitude hormones under stress. By focusing on positive thoughts you can stimulate positive attitude hormones and reprogram the subconscious brain patterns to be more upbeat.

- Take a walk break and recite a mantra. This keeps you under the control of the conscious brain. Verbal statements will activate the logical left side of the frontal lobe to avoid drifting off under the subconscious brain control.

- The mental empowerment of walk breaks. Every week dozens of runners tell me that when they tried to run continuously they became discouraged, often assuming that they were not designed to run. Just the thought that they could walk as desired was the freedom needed to start again.

- Runners like to be in control—Run Walk Run gives you control. You never have to be exhausted from a run. By walking more frequently, you can feel better during the run, recover more quickly, and reduce or eliminate pain. You determine how often to walk and how long to run or walk, and reap the benefits of running without the downsides. Designating the amount of running and the amount of walking, allows you to focus on a running segment that you know you can do.

- Walk breaks allow you to enjoy the endorphins. Physiologists tell us that strenuous activity will trigger the release of endorphins. The primary role of these hormones is to kill pain. Running continuously will irritate certain areas usually producing damage and endorphins. Taking a walk break will stop the continuous stress, allowing the endorphins to perform the secondary role that we love: injecting an attitude boost. Experts believe that endorphins are the most positive of the positive attitude hormones experienced by humans.

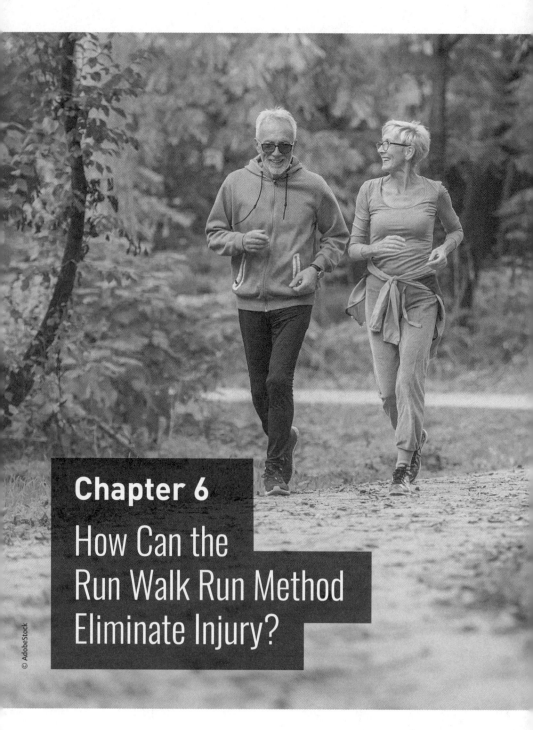

Chapter 6

How Can the Run Walk Run Method Eliminate Injury?

Our bodies are designed to walk for long distances. Running continuously is much more difficult and stressful. Even as we adapt to the running motion, each of us has a few weak links that take on more stress. These are the areas that ache, hurt, or don't work correctly when we run too far or too fast for the current level of fitness. Weak links commonly hurt when we restart our training after some time off, don't provide sufficient rest after a hard workout, or eliminate walk breaks because we feel good.

In some cases, pain-killing hormones, such as endorphins, will mask the damage. Most commonly, exercisers go into denial, ignore the first signs of irritation, and keep training until the stressed area breaks down.

Most of the aches and pains experienced by my runners and walkers are located in these weak link areas—the muscles, joints, tendons, etc. that take more stress due to the individual range of motion, body structure, type of workout, etc. The process starts during a normal workout when micro tears develop in muscles and tendons due to the focused stress of continued movement and irritation of these key parts. The number of these tiny injuries will increase on long or faster workouts, especially during the last third. But in most cases, the rest period after a workout will allow for healing of most or all of this damage.

Walk breaks stop or significantly reduce the continuous buildup of stress on the weak links. By increasing the frequency of the walk breaks and shortening the length of the run segment, most of the runners I've coached, who have been injured, have been able to continue running as the injury healed. Non-stop runners who have had repeat injuries have been amazed at how the strategy of Run Walk Run can prevent future incidents.

The concept is to stay below the threshold of irritation. The most common way to do this is to keep reducing the duration of the run segment, with frequent insertion of walk breaks.

With shorter running segments and longer walks, there is less pain, and the endorphins can inject into receptor sites on billions of cells. This sends a positive attitude boost throughout mind and body.

Run Walk Run is a dynamic system that can be adjusted each day to allow for more healing and to prevent early stage injuries from getting worse. Being sensitive to possible irritation and adjusting the Run Walk Run strategy can speed recovery dramatically from the more strenuous workouts.

As you take action, you shift brain control into the conscious, executive brain, and you can gain major control over your orthopedic health.

Can I run while injured?

Thousands of runners have reported that by using liberal walk breaks, they were able to continue running, while allowing the injury to heal. In some cases, the blood flow generated by walking with gentle and short jog segments has been cited in healing some injuries as opposed to a complete layoff from running.

The following is training advice, given from one runner to another. For medical advice, see a doctor.

1. Choose a doctor who wants you to run in some form, as soon as you can. Explain that you are using the Galloway Run Walk Run method in which very short running segments are gradually introduced into gentle walks. When you find such a doctor, get his or her advice about returning to running. Some injuries, such as stress fractures, will not allow for running for a number of weeks. Consult with your doctor.

2. Most injuries require at least a day or two of no running to get the repair started in the damaged area. Most running injuries I've had have allowed for walking or aqua-jogging. These two exercises can maintain conditioning so that the return to running is easier. Again, check with the doctor to see if these exercises would be appropriate.

3. When given the OK to ease into running, start with 5 sec of running/55 sec of walking. This will maintain most of your running adaptations and has been the most successful strategy for running and healing at the same time. If the injury will not allow for this, go back to walking or take additional days off and treat the injury.

4. Monitor the damaged area as you start back. If the symptoms get worse, stop running for a few days and consult with a doctor.

5. As symptoms decrease, you can either increase distance or increase the amount of running while decreasing the amount of walking. Do so gently.

6. Be prepared to drop back to more walking if symptoms increase again.

Run Walk Run Adjustments to Reduce Irritation:

As long as you have been cleared to do some short runs, here are some adjustments that have allowed runners to continue running during the healing process:
- Used to use 3 min run/1 min walk—shift to 30 sec run/30 sec walk
- Used to use 60/30—substitute 15/15
- Used to use 30/30—substitute 10 sec run/30 sec walk

For a more conservative approach, use the plan in chapter 10.

Note: Read the section on Acceleration Gliders (chapter 13) and do this drill 4-8 times (once or twice a week) to avoid abrupt starting and stopping.

Why do micro tears accumulate?

- Not enough walk breaks
- Run segments are too long
- Constant use
- Prior damage
- Speedwork
- Too many races
- Doing something different

- Sudden increase of workload
- Inadequate rest between workouts
- Not enough walk breaks during runs
- Stretching (yes stretching causes a lot of injuries)
- Heavy body weight

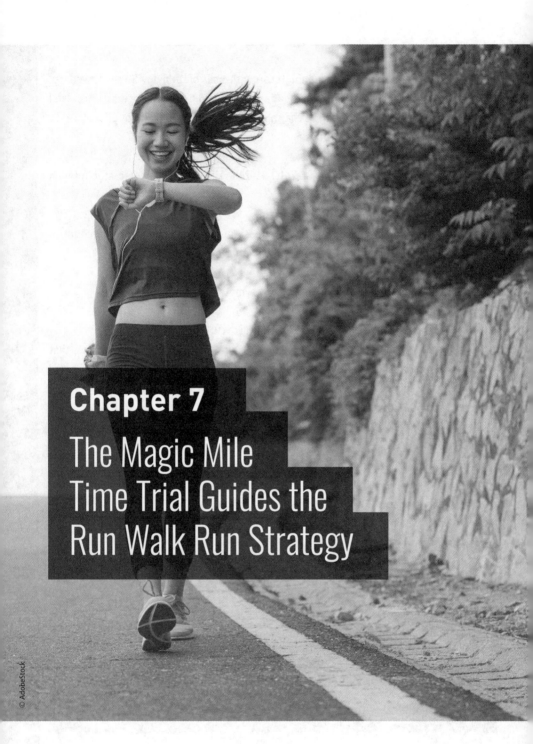

Chapter 7

The Magic Mile
Time Trial Guides the
Run Walk Run Strategy

© AdobeStock

Knowing what a realistic pace for a given run is can indicate the right Run Walk Run strategy. The Magic Mile (MM) can set the pace. This simple cognitive strategy can keep you from setting unrealistic goals and then training too hard. As you do the math you will know current capabilities and how much improvement may be possible during a season. The Run Walk Run strategies are directly linked to the pace per mile.

I've used a number of different evaluation tools over my 50+ years of running. The MM has been the most accurate reality check in setting a safe pace and then a Run Walk Run strategy for all workouts. It will also provide guidance as to when a goal change might be productive. To ensure continued injury-free running enjoyment, you need to know current potential in order to set the right Run Walk Run strategy for various paces. Without the MM, most runners usually set an unrealistic goal, which leads to overtraining and frustration.

NOTE: Beginners should follow the suggestions in chapter 10.

How to do the MM

- These one-mile time trials are listed on the schedules in my books. They are usually run about every 2-3 weeks. Only one MM is done each day it is assigned.

- Go to a track, or other accurately measured course. One mile is 4 laps around a standard track (1600 meters).

- Warm up by walking for 5 minutes, then use a Run Walk Run strategy that is more conservative than you will use in your MM. If you plan to use a 3-minute run/1-minute walk in the MM, then the warm-up ratio would be run a minute and walk a minute, or 30 seconds/30 seconds. Then, for 5-10 minutes, jog at an easy pace, with walk breaks as desired.

- Do 4 acceleration gliders. These are listed in chapter 13.

- Walk for 2-3 minutes.

- On your first MM, don't run all-out from the start—just run a normal pace for 3 laps and then pick it up a little. Be sure to record your time, and try to remember and record the time of each lap

- Try to run faster on each successive MM. Run fast—for you—for 4 laps. It is your choice to either use walk breaks or not during the MM (most of my runners who report times from non-stop vs. Run Walk Run, usually run faster with some form of a walk break in the MM).

- A school track is the best venue. Don't use a treadmill because they tend to be notoriously unreliable, and often tell you that you ran farther or faster than you really did.

- If using a GPS device to measure the mile, use a flat, safe course and measure the same mile several times. Mark the beginning and end based upon the results of 3-4 measurements. Then measure the quarter-mile segments. It's best to use the same segment for each MM.

- On each successive MM, adjust pace in order to run a faster time. Never sprint.

- Cool down by jogging and walking gently for 10 minutes and then walking for 5-10 minutes.

- Use the formula below to see what time is predicted during a season.

- Then use the results to set a realistic pace for the long runs.

- The pace for each run will indicate the appropriate Run Walk Run® strategy—noted in the next chapter.

- Adjust pacing during each quarter mile to help with improvement.

- A good formula for success is to keep a consistent pace for the first 3 quarters with a slightly faster last lap.

- You may run the rest of the miles scheduled for that day at any pace or Run Walk Run strategy.

Note: Remember that you are only running one MM each day it is scheduled.

How to run the MM

On the first MM, run gently for three laps and pick up the pace a bit on the last. Try to remember the time of each quarter mile (one lap around a track is close enough to a quarter mile if you run in the middle of the first lane). On each successive MM afterward, run the first lap slightly slower than you think you can average. Take a short walk break at the quarter mile, half mile, or even eighth mile marks. If you aren't huffing and puffing, you can pick up the pace a bit on the second lap. If you are huffing after the first lap, then just hold your pace on lap two—or reduce it slightly.

Walk breaks during a MM? Many runners find that they run faster when they insert a 15- to 30-second walk break every half lap or every lap or at least at the half mile. At the end of lap 3, the walk break is optional. It is OK to be breathing hard on the last lap. If you are slowing down on the last lap, start a little slower on the next MM. When you finish, you should feel like you couldn't run more than about half a lap at that pace. You may find that you don't need many (or any) walk breaks during the MM—experiment and adjust.

Don't Sprint!

How hard should I run the MM?

The first one should be only slightly faster than you normally run. With each successive MM, pick up the pace and try to beat your previous best time. By the fourth MM, you should be running fairly close to your potential.

Should I use walk breaks during the MM?

Most of the runners I've coached who have tried both non-stop running and Run Walk Run have reported faster times when walk breaks were inserted in some form. Try it both ways.

Galloway's Performance Predictor

Step 1:   Run your MM time trial (4 laps around the track or 1,600 meters).

Step 2:   Convert the MM time to minutes and hundredths of a minute (9:33 MM is 9.55).

Step 3:   Compute your current potential mile pace for the race of your choice by using the following formula.

Step 4:   Compute the pace of long runs by adding 2 minutes to the potential marathon pace.

Step 5:   Do the training necessary to prepare for the goal of your choice

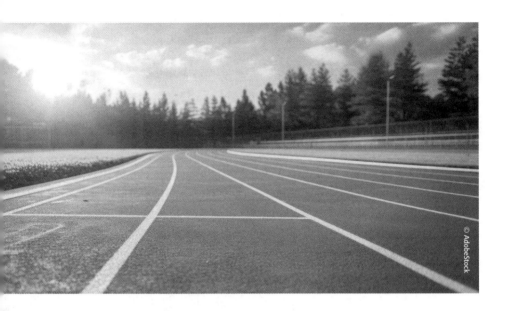

© AdobeStock

Using periodic MMs to predict best potential per mile in a race

- 5K—add 33 seconds to the best current MM
- 10K—multiply by 1.15
- Half Marathon—multiply by 1.2
- Marathon—multiply by 1.3

Example: Magic Mile time: 10:00

5K potential pace per mile: 10 + 33 seconds = 10:33 per mile

10K potential per mile pace: multiply 10 x 1.15 = 11:30 per mile

Half marathon potential per mile pace: multiply 10 x 1.2 = 12 min/mi

Marathon potential per mile pace: Multiply 10 x 1.3 = 13 min/mi

Long run training pace: add 2 minutes per mile = 15 minutes per mile

Note: Slow down the long runs and long races by 30 sec/mile for every 5°F increase above 60°F (20 sec/km for every 2°C above 14°C).

Metric runners: multiply the mile pace by .62 to determine pace per kilometer

Note: The potential that is determined by the computations assumes that you will be running about all-out effort in your goal race, that you did all of the training in my time goal programs, and that conditions were perfect on race day. Because conditions are not usually perfect it is best to add a few seconds per mile to what the MM predicts on a perfect day, for at least the first few miles of your goal race.

First-time racers should run to finish only

I strongly recommend that first-time runners in any race should not attempt a time goal. Use the MM to determine your long run pace (adding 2 minutes to the MM time multiplied by 1.3). During the race itself, I recommend running the first two-thirds of the race at your training pace. During the last third you may run as you wish.

Time goal runners may make a "leap of faith" goal prediction

I have no problem at the beginning of a training season allowing my e-coach athletes, who've run one or more races at a certain distance, to choose a goal time that is faster than that predicted by the initial MM in the same race. As you do the speed training, the long runs and your form drills, most runners improve...but how much? In my experience this leap-of-faith goal should not exceed 3-5% improvement in a 6-month training program.

How to set up the leap of faith

- Run the MM

- Use the formula above to predict your current potential per mile pace in your goal race

- Choose the amount of improvement during the training program (3-5%)

Example: "leap of faith" improvement in a half marathon

Half-Marathon Pre-test prediction	3% Improvement	5% Improvement
1:20	2:12	4:00
1:40	3:00	5:00
2:00	3:36	6:00
2:30	4:30	7:30
3:00	5:24	9:00

(Over a 4-6 month training program)

The key to goal setting is keeping your ego in check. From my experience, I have found that a 3% improvement is realistic. This means that if your half-marathon time is predicted to be 3:00, then it is realistic to assume you could lower it by five and a half minutes if you do the speed training and the long runs as noted on my training schedules in my books. The maximum improvement, which is less likely, is a more aggressive 5% or 9 minutes off a three-hour half marathon.

In both of these situations, however, everything must come together to produce the predicted result. Even runners who shoot for a 3% improvement and do all the training as described, achieve their goal slightly more than 50% of the time during a racing season. The more aggressive performances usually result in success about 20% of the time. There are many factors that determine a time goal in any race that are outside of your control: weather, terrain, infection, etc.

The prediction from the MM assumes that you have done all of the training for the goal (e.g., long runs and speed workouts), the weather is ideal, the course is not hilly, and that you don't have to weave around runners very much—or swing wide around too many turns.

Note: Crowded races force you to run longer than race distance—usually about half a mile in a half marathon and one mile additional in a marathon.

MM time trials give you a reality check throughout the program

- Follow the same format as listed in the pre-test above.

- By doing this as noted, you will learn how to pace yourself.

- Hint: It's better to start a bit more slowly than you think you can run.

- Walk breaks will be helpful for most runners. Read chapter 8 for suggested ratios.

- Note whether you are speeding up or slowing down at the end, and adjust in the next MM.

- If you are not making progress then look for reasons and take action.

Reasons why you may not be improving:

- You're overtrained, and tired—if so, reduce your training, or take an extra rest day.

- You may have chosen a goal that is too ambitious for your current ability.

- You may have missed some of your workouts, or not been as regular with your training as needed.

- The temperature may have been above 60°F (14°C). Temperatures above 60°F will cause a slowdown (the longer the race, the more time added).

- You ran the first or second lap too fast.

Final reality check

Time-goal runners: Take your fastest MM and use Galloway's Performance Predictor above. It is recommended that you run the first third of your goal race a few seconds per mile slower than the pace predicted by the MM.

To-finish runners should run the first two-thirds of the race at training pace and then speed up if desired.

If the MMs are predicting a time that is slower than the goal you've been training for, go with the time predicted by the MM.

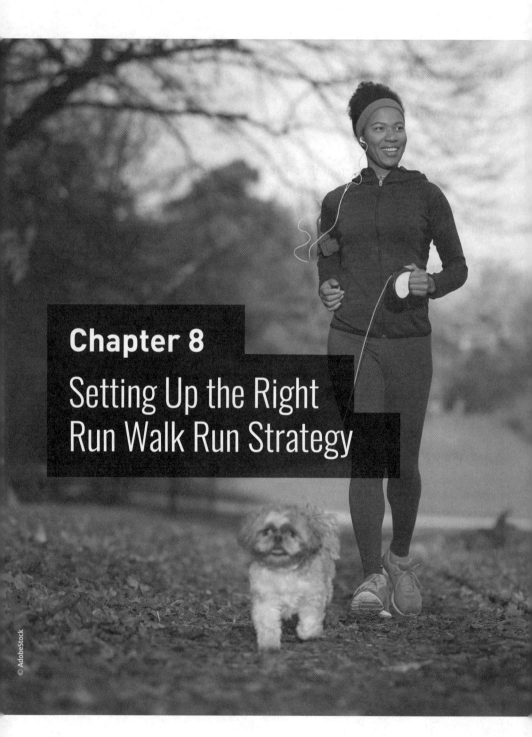

Chapter 8

Setting Up the Right Run Walk Run Strategy

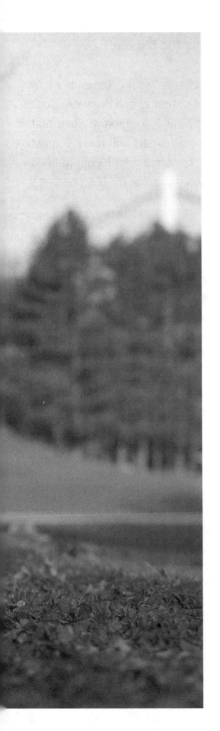

In the previous chapter you learned how to predict current potential, and how realistic a leap-of-faith performance improvement may be. By using the Magic Mile (MM) one can also set a safe pace for long runs by adding two minutes to the current marathon potential pace. In this chapter you will see my recommendations for the specific strategies of Run Walk Run (RWR)—based on specific paces.

Be sure to follow the heat slowdown rule: 30 seconds per mile slower for every 5°F increase above 60°F (20 sec/km slower for every 2°C above 14°C).

Once you have set the appropriate pace—whether long run, race, or regular workout—one can use the strategies below, based upon the pace that is used at that time. There are special rules that apply to short races, such as one mile, 5K, and 10K.

You cannot run too slowly on long runs

Beginners should read chapter 10 before reading this chapter. The general rule during the first year of running is that you cannot go too slow or walk too often. Goal one is to stay injury free. Goal two is to enjoy every run. The best way I've found to reach these goals is to walk early and often.

How to set up the right Run Walk Run strategy for the day

- Use the MM to calculate pace. Go over the last chapter again. Remember that the first MM should be gentle—as an introduction to timing and distance—don't run this initial one fast! The goal on subsequent MMs is to improve upon that time. In the beginning of a training program, most runners will make a great deal of progress, but don't worry if you don't. It takes some a lot longer to build a performance base than others. Patience is not only a virtue for beginners—it's a strategy.

- First priority—whether seasoned veteran or new beginner—is setting the right pace for long runs. Even if your MM time is slower than you know you can run for one mile, do the math. There is no liability on long runs, for any runner, in pacing the long ones too slow or taking too many walk breaks.

- Set up the Run Walk Run strategy based upon the pace per mile, as noted below. On long runs—marathons and half marathons—the ratios below can be directly applied.

- If you want to walk more frequently on long runs—do it! Injury risk will drop and recovery will be faster with shorter run segments and more frequent walks.

- Beginners can use the ratios below for all races and all training runs.

- Veterans can use some variations on shorter distance races and runs, by practicing various ratios at goal pace to see what works best. These race rehearsal segments are run during a short run day, during the week.

Run Walk Run Strategies

After having heard back from over 500,000 runners who have used walk breaks at various paces, I've come up with the following suggested ratios. As mentioned, these are strategies and can be adjusted as desired by individuals.

Note: 30 seconds has been found to be the longest effective walk break at paces of 9 min/mile and slower.

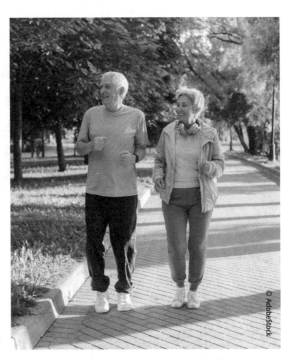

Reports from thousands of runners who have used variations between 20 seconds and 60 seconds tend to show that most receive as much recovery from a 20- to 30-second walk break as from a longer walk. So by shortening both the run segment and the walk segment, there is often less fatigue at the end.

In fact, there is a slowdown during the second 30 seconds of a 60-second walk break. This makes it harder and harder to start up after a walk break at the end of a long run or long race.

Strategies

Pace/mile	Run	Walk
7:00	6 min	30 sec (or run one mile/walk 40 seconds)
7:30	5 min	30 sec (or 2:30/15)
8:00	4 min	30 sec (or 2/15)
8:30	3 min	30 sec (or 2/23)
9:00	2 min	30 sec or 80/20
9:30 -10:45	R90sec/W30sec or R60sec/W20sec or R45sec/W15sec or R60sec/W30sec or R40sec/W20sec	
10:45-12:15	R60sec/W30sec or R40sec/W20sec or R30sec/W15sec or R30sec/W30sec or R20sec/W20sec	
12:15-14:30	R30sec/W30sec or R20sec/W20sec or R15sec/W15sec	
14:30-15:45	R15sec/W30sec	
15:45-17:00	R10sec/W30sec	
17:00-18:30	R8sec/W30sec or R5sec/W25sec or R10sec/W30sec	
18:30-20:00	R5sec/W30sec or R5sec/W25sec or R4sec/W30sec	

R3min/W30sec = Run 3 minutes/Walk 30 seconds

You may always divide each of the amounts by 2 or 3.

Years ago, runners were running 9-min/mile pace using R4min/W1min. After working with thousands at that pace we've found it better to run for 2 minutes and walk for 30 seconds; R80sec/W20sec; or R60sec/W15sec.

Instead of running a 12-minute pace using R2min/W1min, you could use R60sec/ W30sec; R40sec/W20sec; or R30sec/W15sec.

Instead of running a 13-min/mile pace using R1min/W1min, you can use R30sec/ W30sec; R20sec/W20sec; R15sec/W15sec; or R10sec/W10 sec.

Be sure to adjust for heat.

Walk more going uphill—the "huff and puff" rule

If you are running a 10-min/mile pace on flat ground, your pace should slow to 11 min/mile or 12 min/mile going up a moderate-grade hill and the ratio should be adjusted accordingly as noted above. There are many individual issues when running uphill or at higher elevations. The best and simplest rule when running uphill is to avoid huffing and puffing. If you start to increase respiration from that on the flat sections, slow down and take more frequent walk breaks immediately.

Other modifications

Downhill. Those who use efficient downhill running form (feet low to the ground, light touch of the feet, moderate or shorter stride) can often run for longer segments going down. This type of running form uses the ankle, reducing or eliminating aggravation on the knees and other joints. Pounding on the feet and shins can be taken away by using this technique.

Walk breaks on shorter distance races: 5K, 10K, 10 mile. The ratios listed above have been proven to improve finish times in half and full marathons. I recommend that some race rehearsal segments be done during one of the short distance runs each week. After a warm-up, run 4 to 6 half-mile segments at race pace with a 2- to 3-minute walk break between each. During each half-mile segment (2 laps around a track) try a different strategy to find which feels best and works best.

On shorter distance races, the amounts can be adjusted for the individual. Here are some suggestions:

Strategy in Half/Marathon	5K	10K	10 mile
9 min/mi	R3min/W20-30sec	R3min/W30sec	R2:30min/W30sec
10 min/mi	R3min/W30sec	R2:30min/W30sec	R2min/W30sec
11-12 min/mi	R90/W30sec	R80min/W30sec	R60min/W30sec
13-14 min/mi	R40/W30sec	R30/W20 sec	R30/W25sec

R3min/W30sec = Run 3 minutes/Walk 30 seconds

When can I reduce or stop taking walk breaks in races? I recommend waiting until the last third of the race to cut down or eliminate walk breaks. Prepare for this by running continuously for the last 1-2 miles of some of your short runs.

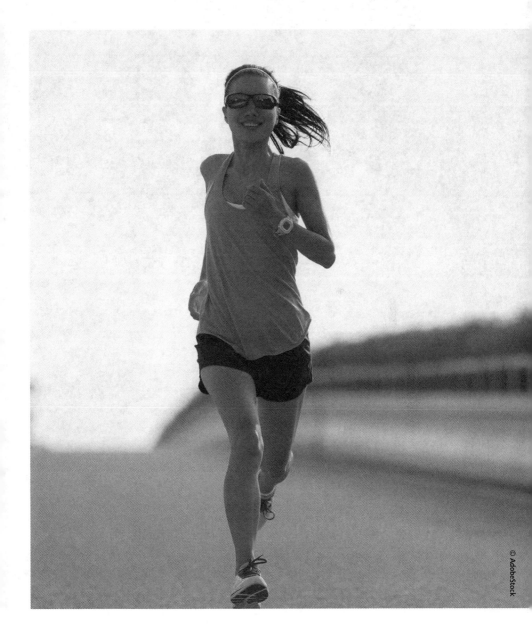

© AdobeStock

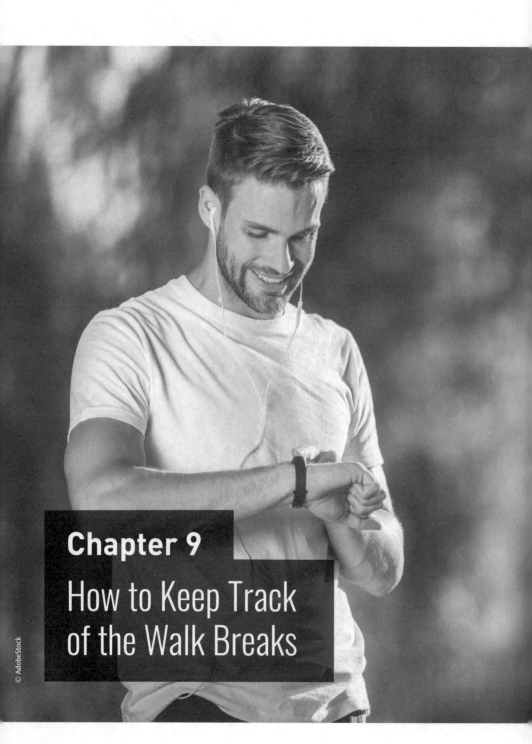

Chapter 9

How to Keep Track of the Walk Breaks

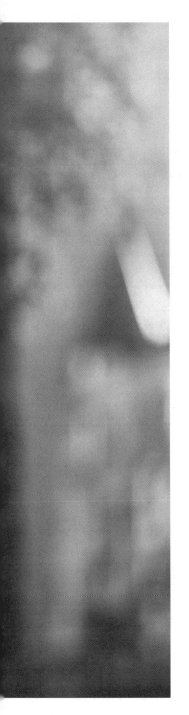

Runners who used to feel a distracting interruption when trying to manually time their walk breaks have smartwatch timers or my Galloway Run Walk Run app help them ease into a new rhythm. Here are some of the timing options.

You can become like Pavlov's dog. Runners tell me that they get into a rhythm as they follow the beep. After a few weeks using a set amount of running and walking, you can hardwire this behavior pattern into your subconscious brain. Such patterns tend to become somewhat automatic as you use the ratio regularly.

The best option is my Run Walk Run app, available in the app store. The app makes it easy to track your run and walk intervals on your smartphone or smartwatch.

Of course, all smartphones and smartwatches come with options for tracking your workouts. You can also find various apps for interval training that will allow you to track your run and walk intervals and keep track of your total workout time.

Use a timer!

- Timers can reprogram the subconscious brain. You don't have to guess or look at your watch all the time—just listen for the beep.

- The little green coach. A runner was using our green Galloway timer in a race. At first, he would catch up with a group of runners during his run, walk at the beep as they ran (non-stop) ahead. After the half-way point, he moved steadily ahead of this group as their fatigue produced a slowdown. As he was enjoying the after race refreshments, they finished, recognized him and said "Tell me about your little green coach."

- Apps and other tools that deliver the walk-break prompts. There are several apps by Iolofit that allow you to set the run-walk ratio of choice, with music in the background. I have recorded the coaching advice for each workout with some motivation in training for 5K, 10K, half marathon, and marathon. Choose the "Galloway Ultimate" label for these apps. Among the innovations is the increase in the beat of the music as you pick up the pace.

- One of the benefits of wearing the timer in a race is that the beep will warn other runners near you as you move to the side of the road to take walk breaks. In the beginning of a race, some runners like to use 5 beeps, and then change to 2 beeps later in the race.

- When running in quiet surroundings or in nature you can use the vibration mode— no sound.

The mystery beeper story

I was running in a wooded area on a beautiful morning in Springfield MO, using my timer on the beep mode. After about 10 minutes, I heard another beep nearby, just after each of my beeps. I looked around but didn't see anyone. Over the next 5 minutes the sound of the mystery beeper became getting louder, so I stopped and finally identified the source: a mockingbird in a nearby tree.

How to set up the Galloway timer

1. Insert a AAA battery in the back.

2. Hold the timer so that you are looking at the screen.

3. Turn on the timer by touching the middle indention on the top of the timer

4. Push the middle indention again to change the first field (the run portion). The digits will blink. Hit the right button on the top of the timer to lower the amount and touch the left button on the top to increase the amount of time. When you have the right amount for the run, hit the middle indention again to move to the walk amount and set it the same way.

5. Hit the middle indention on the top again to move to the interval amount. Hit the right button on top to get "99."

6. Then hit the center indention again to set the vibrate or beep mode. Finally set the number of beeps or vibrations.

7. Turn off the timer by holding the middle indention down for a few seconds until the screen goes blank.

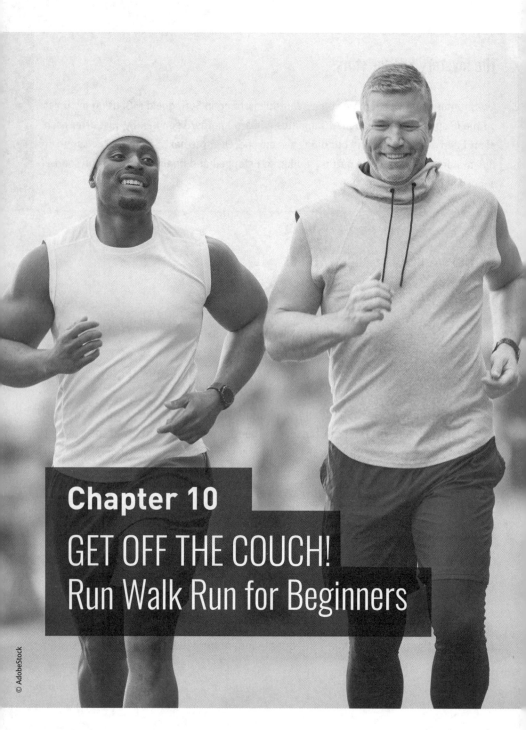

Chapter 10

GET OFF THE COUCH!
Run Walk Run for Beginners

© AdobeStock

I've personally heard from tens of thousands of runners who said my Run Walk Run method was the only thing that got them running. When you reduce the amount of running enough, with the right amount of gentle walking to recover, almost anyone can run without aches, pains, or debilitating fatigue.

The human body has evolved as an extremely efficient walking machine. Running requires a lot more resources and builds up stress on the system and on weak links. One anthropologist who studies ancient man told me that we were probably designed to run non-stop for about 200 yards—to get away from predators, jump over obstacles, etc. We can adapt to run very long distances—but at a great cost: dramatic increase in energy reserves, pounding of body weight on feet and joints, increase in core body temperature, and much quicker muscle exhaustion.

When strategic walk breaks are taken from the beginning of a run and in the right ratio for the individual, the legs, feet, and joints can continuously adapt. Fatigue is erased, energy resources are conserved, body temperature is managed, and weak links don't get overused.

The Run Walk Run method is a cognitive strategy

As you focus on each segment of running and then each segment of walking you activate the conscious brain. This allows you to gain control over the emotional subconscious brain, and activate positive attitude hormones.

Change somebody's life for the better!

Thousands of veteran runners have mentored beginners into running by using this method. By encouraging a novice to use this program, you can improve the quality of life: better attitude, more vitality, more focus, etc. Not many people have the opportunity to improve the quality of someone's life—it is empowering.

• Run Walk Run bestows the same joy of running as derived from running non-stop for almost everyone who has reported on this.

- The right formula of Run Walk Run has allowed older or heavier runners to start running for the first time in their lives without pain—and continue to improve and increase distance.

- Many of these challenged runners have been able to finish half marathons or marathons within 6-9 months of taking their first steps.

- The sixth edition of my book *Running: Getting Started* (March 2024) is a good training resource for beginners. It has a 6-month program with support information for beginners (available autographed from *www.JeffGalloway.com*).

Goals produce results

When beginners have a goal written on a calendar, they are more likely to stay motivated and get in the workouts that transform body and mind into an active, positive organism. Goals activate the executive brain that can override the subconscious emotional brain when one is not motivated or is under stress. At the end of this chapter you'll find a 5K training program that has been very successful in not only getting runners and walkers across the finish line but also the line from sedentary to active.

How to start: A 20-step program

1. There is no one pattern for everyone. Each was born with different abilities and weak links. Don't try to keep up with a friend when you are feeling significant fatigue or pain.

2. Walk first! Gradually increase the length of a gentle walk to 30 minutes.

3. Whether walking or running, use a relatively short, gentle stride.

4. When starting to run, walk gently for 10 minutes at the beginning and the end of your Run Walk Run segment.

5. On the first day of running, run gently for 5 seconds and then walk for the rest of the minute. If there are no problems, continue alternating 5 seconds of running with 55 seconds of walking for 5-10 minutes.

6. Use a running stride that is short, with the feet low to the ground and a light touch of the foot. This is sometimes called the shuffle. For more information, see chapter 11 on running form.

7. NO HUFFING AND PUFFING! Slow down and walk more to breathe normally.

8. Take a day off before you do the Run Walk Run again. Gentle walking on this off day is generally OK.

9. It's important to do the Run Walk Run, in some form, every other day if you want to maintain the adaptations of running.

10. During each successive Run Walk Run workout, continue to use R5sec/W55sec and increase by 3-4 additional minutes until you reach 30 minutes.

11. If desired, reduce the walk warm-up and warm-down to 5 minutes each.

12. Some may want to stay at R5sec/W55sec—and this is fine. Most beginners maintain this strategy for 2-3 weeks.

13. To increase the running portion, do R5sec/W55sec for the first 20 minutes and then shift to R10sec/W50sec for the last 5-10 minutes of the workout.

14. To continue shifting to the R10sec/W50sec, gradually add 3-4 minutes of this ratio to the end of each workout, while decreasing the same amount of minutes of R5sec/W55sec, until you are doing 30 minutes of R10sec/W50sec.

15. There is no goal for reaching any specific ratio in any specific period of time. Each person can decide how much to run and how much to walk on any given day.

16. One can continue to move up to R15sec/W45sec, R20sec/W40sec, R30sec/ W30sec, or any ratio that is comfortable by gradually increasing as noted above.

17. If you are huffing and puffing—even at the end of a workout—you either ran too fast or increased the running portions too quickly. Back off a little bit.

18. Don't hesitate to drop back to an easier ratio if you are not feeling good on a given day. On some days you will need to do this. It is part of the running experience to gain control over your attitude, aches, etc. by walking more and running less on those days.

19. Enjoy every run. If you are not feeling good, take a 2- to 3-minute gentle walk to catch up, and walk more and run less for the rest of the run.

20. Smile and enjoy every endorphin.

Getting started 5K training program

Time required: 30 minutes on two weekdays (Tue/Thu or Mon/Wed) plus one weekend Run Walk Run that will build gradually to 3.5 miles.

Who: This program is designed for those who are just beginning to increase distance, those making a comeback after a period of inactivity, etc. The advice is given as one exerciser to another. For medical issues, see a doctor.

Textbook: My book, *Galloway's 5K/10K Running*, has additional information for both of these events. You can order this book from *www.jeffgalloway.com*.

Use a short stride: Whether walking or running, adjust your stride so that it is relaxed and well within a natural range of motion for you. Keep the feet low to the ground. Shorter strides reduce effort and orthopedic stress, allowing the body to adapt naturally to running and walking.

The long one: As you increase the length of the long run every two weeks, you'll extend endurance limits, improve mental concentration at the end of workouts, and enhance your physiological infrastructure. Longer workouts improve your cardiovascular plumbing system so that you can deliver blood better to the exercising muscles and withdraw waste more effectively. The endurance workout is the primary training component in a 5K program.

Mental focus: As you focus on each workout, your goal on the calendar, and each run and walk segment, you shift mental control into the conscious brain. This overrides the subconscious, emotional brain that will trigger negative attitude hormones under stress.

How to determine pace per mile: Use the Magic Mile (MM) as noted in chapter 7.

Example:

MM was 10:00.
Multiply by 1.3 = 13:00
Add 2 minutes = 15 min/mi on long runs.

Note: Slow the pace down by 30 sec/mile for every 5-degree temperature increase above 60°F (slow down by 20 sec/km for every 2°C above 14°C) on long runs.

Maintenance workouts: Usually, the long workout is done on weekends, and the two maintenance workouts are done during the week. The pace of these can be as slow or as fast as you want to go, as long as you are recovering well from the weekend long ones. Beware of fast running as this increases the risk of aches, pains, and injuries.

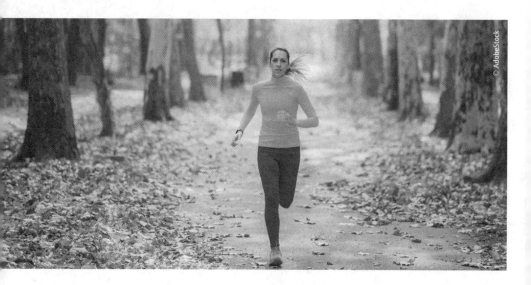

Rest days: When you go farther than you have gone before, your muscles, tendons, joints, etc. need a recovery period to rebuild stronger. Take the day off from exercise the day before and the day after a long one. On the other non-running days, you can do any exercise that does not fatigue the calf muscle. Walking, aqua-jogging, swimming, cycling, elliptical work, and rowing are fine, but stair machines, lower body strength training, and step aerobics are not.

Warm-up: Walk for 3 minutes, then run for 5-10 seconds and walk for the rest of the minute for 10 minutes. Then use the Run Walk Run® ratio that is appropriate.

Cool-down: After your workout, don't stop. Walk gently for the next 10 minutes. You're done!:

If you are already running more than 1.5 miles, you can start at the length of the long run which matches your current long-run distance during the past 2 weeks in the following training schedule.

Note: At *www.JeffGalloway.com* you can find a timer that will beep or vibrate to tell you when to walk and when to run.

The schedule:

Week	Tuesday	Thursday	Saturday
1	10 min	13 min	1.5 miles (2.5 km)
2	16 min	19 min	30 min
3	22 min	25 min	2 miles (3.3 km)
4	28 min	30 min	30 min
5	30 min	30 min	2.5 miles (4 km)
6	30 min	30 min	30 min (800T)
7	30 min	30 min	3 miles (5 km)
8	30 min	30 min	40 min
9	30 min	30 min	3.5 miles (5.8 km)
10	30 min	30 min	30 min
11	30 min	30 min	5K race
12	30 min	30 min	30 min
13	30 min	30 min	3-3.5 miles (on to the next goal!)

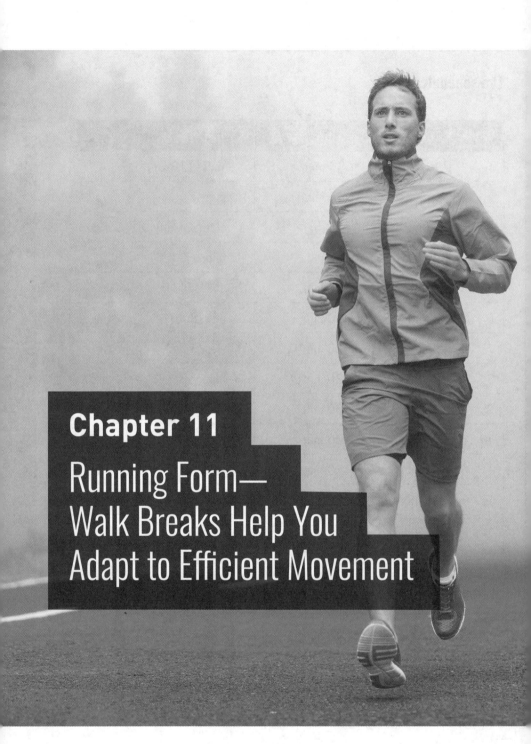

Chapter 11

Running Form—
Walk Breaks Help You
Adapt to Efficient Movement

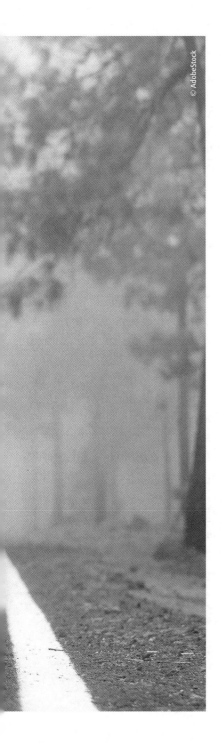

© AdobeStock

My experience in doing running form evaluations for over 10,000 runners, backed by research, is that your body will naturally adapt to an efficient motion if you run naturally. This means that you should not try to run the way someone else runs, or force yourself to run in a way that is not natural.

Strategic walk breaks will help your body make a form efficiency adjustment. Extra walk breaks can often allow for adaptations to avoid aches or pains. When the walk breaks are made often enough from the beginning, you can reduce the normal fatigue buildup. Each walk break allows you the conscious opportunity to monitor the continuous buildup of stress on foot, leg, muscle, joint, etc. If there are problems during the walk you can adjust stride, foot placement, posture, and walk-break ratio to stay energized without pain.

Posture

Most runners I've worked with run better and reduce pain by running upright: head over shoulders, over hips as you touch the ground. But if you are one of the few that naturally lean forward when walking or running (and don't have back or neck pain) you should run the natural way for you. Back and neck pain are often decreased significantly when one maintains an upright posture.

Good running posture: Visualize that you are a puppet on a string.

Efficient running: Keep your feet low to the ground with a short stride and a light touch.

Stay low to the ground: This allows the ankle to do most of the work, significantly reducing muscle fatigue. When the ankle is the primary running mechanical component, wear and tear on knees and hips can be reduced significantly. Muscle fatigue is also reduced.

Shuffle: The resulting running motion is a shuffle. The ankle is an amazingly efficient lever that can keep you running forward with little effort. A shorter stride with the feet directly underneath stimulates a reflex action in the ankle with consistent propulsion.

Stride: A short but natural stride also activates the ankle, significantly reducing aggravation on other orthopedic units. When the ankle is the primary mechanical component, wear and tear on knees and hips can be reduced significantly.

A stride that is too long: Most of the aches, pains, and even injuries that result from the mechanics of running, have, in my experience, occurred due to a stride that is extended beyond one's natural range of motion. Biomechanical studies show that as runners get faster, the stride shortens. Reducing stride slightly, with feet directly underneath, stimulates a reflex action in the ankle with consistent propulsion. This allows the body to keep adapting as you move forward.

Feet and legs low to the ground: The more you lift your legs off the ground, the more effort required and the greater the chance for aches and pains. Again, a natural and efficient motion of the feet can reduce exertion, allow for better recovery between run segments and let the body adapt and repair. You'll also find it easier to transition between running and walking.

Light touch of the feet: Some people naturally run with a hard pounding motion. If this is not causing aches and pains, natural motion can prevail. But if you are experiencing any aggravations that could be linked to the heavy foot landing, work on a lighter touch. This is usually associated with a shorter stride, with feet low to the running surface. Those who make some pounding noise during a run can try to improve by doing this drill: During a 30-second segment of a run, listen to the sound of your feet for the first ten seconds. During the next twenty seconds try to reduce the volume by making form adjustments. Between each noise reduction segment, walk normally. Do four to eight of these during one or two runs a week.

No aches and pains: As your body adapts to a smoother running form using the right Run Walk Run ratio, aches and pains are reduced and often go away. Walk breaks stop the cycle of stress on the weak links and speed recovery. If you experience an increase in aches, pains, or fatigue, drop back to shorter run segments and more walking.

Ease into a walk break, and then ease back into the run segment: In chapter 13, you'll discover two simple exercises that can help you run more efficiently and smoothly. You'll naturally transition into each walk break and then gradually get the body running again. This will further reduce the chance of aches, pains, and injuries.

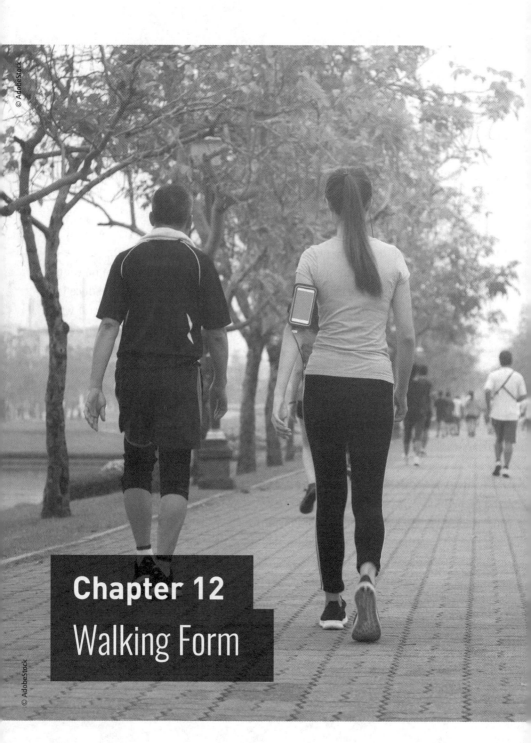

Chapter 12
Walking Form

Most of us have a very efficient walking motion. The subconscious brain intuitively fine-tunes the motion of feet and legs to a range of motion that minimizes effort and energy. Over time, the walking motion becomes more and more efficient, reducing aches and pains.

The best walking form for most of those I've coached is that which is natural to each. Indeed, most of the walking form problems I have seen are experienced by those who try to walk like someone else, or keep up with a walking companion especially when he or she has a longer stride.

Shuffle breaks: Those who start walking or running after years of a very sedentary life should insert some shuffle breaks into their longer walks. Every 3-5 minutes, reduce your walking stride length to baby steps for 30-60 seconds. These strategic recovery breaks will reduce the constant use of the same muscles releasing stress on weak links.

As with walk breaks for runners, each shuffle break allows you to take conscious control over your fatigue and aches at any time—and make walking form adjustments. Go through a short checklist to monitor weak links, overall fatigue, and mechanical issues with the goal of a natural range of motion. Do a periodic form check during each shuffle break using the following principles.

Posture: Most people walk efficiently when in the upright position: head over shoulders over hips as you touch the ground. But as in running, if you are one of the few that naturally lean forward when walking (and don't have back or neck pain) you should walk in the way that feels natural for you. Back and neck pain are often decreased significantly when one maintains an upright posture.

Efficient walking: Use a short and natural stride with your feet and legs low to the ground and with a light touch.

Stride: As in running, a short but natural stride allows the ankle to do most of the work, significantly reducing muscle fatigue. When the ankle is the primary mechanical component, wear and tear on knees and hips can be reduced significantly.

A stride that is too long: In my experience, most of the aches, pains, and even injuries that result from walking occur due to a stride that is extended beyond one's natural range of motion. Shortening the stride with feet directly underneath stimulates a reflex action in the ankle with consistent propulsion. This allows the body to keep adapting as you walk forward.

Feet and legs low to the ground: The more you lift your legs off the ground, the more effort is required and the greater the chance for aches and pains. Again, a natural and efficient motion of the feet can reduce exertion, allow for better recovery between run segments, and let the body adapt and repair.

Light touch of the feet: Some people naturally walk with a hard pounding motion. If this is not causing aches and pains, natural motion can prevail. But if you are

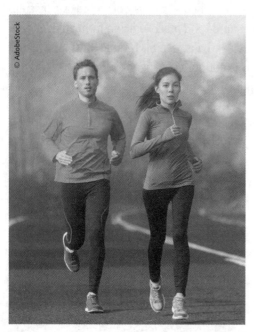

experiencing any aggravations that could be linked to the heavy foot landing, work on a lighter touch. This is usually associated with a shorter stride. Those who make some pounding noise during a walk can usually improve by doing this drill: During a 30-second segment of a walk, listen to the sound of your feet for the first 10 seconds. During the next 20 seconds try to reduce the volume by making form adjustments. Between each noise-reduction segment, walk normally. Do four to eight of these during one or two walks a week.

How to walk faster: Many of my clients have improved the pace of their walk through practice.

Here is the procedure:

1. Follow this routine during the middle of a recovery walk day between runs or during the warm-down walk on a running day.

2. Warm up by walking very gently for at least 5 minutes, then do the following drill.

3. For 10-20 seconds, pick up the cadence of the walk by shortening your stride.

4. Walk gently for 30 seconds

5. Keep alternating segments, finding a cadence or rhythm that is quicker.

6. Ease back on the cadence if you lose smoothness.

7. On the first day, do this for ten minutes.

8. Increase the amount of time you do the alternating segments by 3-4 minutes on each successive session.

9. The goal is to have 20-30 minutes total in this workout.

10. Do this once or twice a week to maintain adaptations.

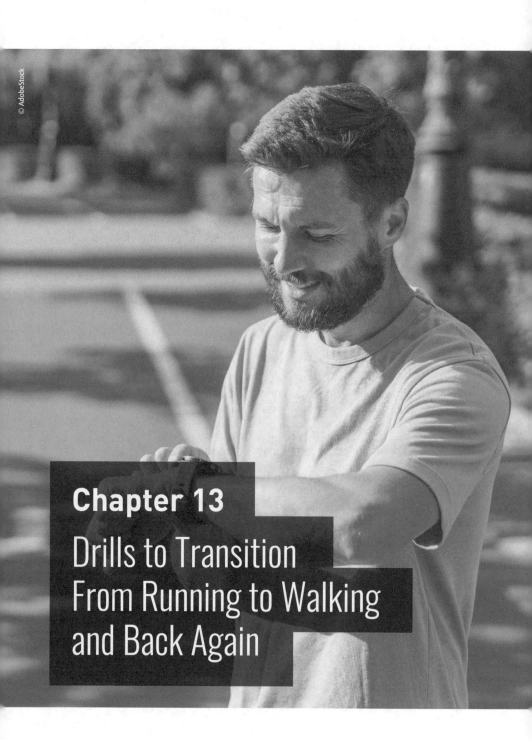

Chapter 13

Drills to Transition From Running to Walking and Back Again

The following gentle drills, which are used at my beach retreats and other individualized sessions, have helped thousands to run faster and more efficiently. They can also help you develop an efficient technique for easing into a walk break and easing into the run segment.

Each targets a few key capabilities. When you put all of them together, your running and walking motions are smoother and more efficient, and times are often faster in races. The drills also help you run lighter on your feet, while strengthening key muscle groups. When runners do these regularly, I've seen significant reduction of excess motion in feet and legs, with reduced impact. Running is easier when you run more smoothly, and the improved cadence of your feet and legs can also result in faster running.

The drills will stimulate activity in the conscious, executive brain. This will keep you focused on the task and exercise control over the emotional, subconscious reflex brain.

When?

These should be done on a non-long-run day. It is fine, however, to do them as part of your warm-up and before a race, an MM, or a speed workout. Many runners have also told me that the drills are a nice way to break up an average run they sometimes call boring. To receive continuing benefits they must be done once or twice every week.

CADENCE DRILL (CD)

Everyone can benefit from doing the CD because it helps to pull all the elements of good running form together at the same time. The CD rewards you for finding an efficient but shorter stride with feet directly underneath the body. This makes it easy to transition into a walk break.

Over the weeks and months, if you do this drill once every week, you will find that your normal cadence slowly increases, naturally. During this drill you are shifting control into the conscious brain—counting, adjusting, and empowering the right side of this frontal lobe to find more efficient ways of running and easing into the walk.

Note: My Run Walk Run app is specifically designed to track intervals and could be used to simplify timing for this drill.

- Warm up by walking for 5 minutes, and then running and walking very gently for 10 minutes.

- Start jogging slowly for 1-2 minutes, and then time yourself for 30 seconds. During these 30 seconds, count the number of times your left or right foot touches (not both).

- At the end of the 30-second interval ease into a walk for about 30 seconds.

- On the second 30-second drill, increase the count by 1 or 2.

- Repeat this 3-7 times. On each successive CD, try to increase by 1-2 additional steps.

- If you reach a count that you can't exceed, just try to maintain the previous count with a smooth motion.

- Start each new CD with a blank slate. Whatever your count on the first one, just try to do more on the second.

In the process of improving cadence, the right side of the conscious brain coordinates a series of adaptations which help the feet, legs, nervous system, and timing mechanism work together as an efficient team:

- Your foot touches more gently.

- Extra, inefficient motions of the foot and leg are reduced or eliminated.

- Less effort is spent on pushing up or moving forward.

- You stay lower to the ground.

- The ankle does most of the work, reducing leg muscle fatigue.

- Your run will glide naturally into a walk.

ACCELERATION-GLIDER DRILLS (AG)

This is another cognitive drill that keeps you focused on each component of running form. By using it 1 or 2 times every week, you develop a range of speeds, with the muscle conditioning to move smoothly from one to the next. The greatest benefit comes as you learn how to glide, or coast off your momentum directly into a walk break.

- Do the AG on a non-long-run day, in the middle of a shorter run, or as a warm-up for a speed session, race, or MM.

- Warm up with at least half a mile of easy running.

- Many runners do the CD just after the easy warm-up, and then the AGs, but the drills can be done separately also.

- Run 4-8 of them.

- Do this at least once a week.

- No sprinting! Never run all-out.

- Don't do these if you have an injury.

- Stop immediately if you suspect that you are irritating a weak link.

After teaching this drill at my one-day running schools and weekend retreats for years, I can say that most people learn better through practice when they work on the concepts listed below—rather than the details—of the drill. So just get out there and try them! The glide segment of this drill has been the best way I've found to train someone to move efficiently from a run into a walk break.

Gliding—This is the most important concept. It is like coasting off the momentum of a downhill run. You can do some of your gliders running down a hill if you want, but it is important to do at least two of them on the flat land. Your goal is to use your momentum, if only for 5-10 strides, gliding smoothly into a walk break.

Do this every week—As with the CDs, it's important to do them 1 or 2 times a week. If you're like most runners, you won't glide very far at first. Regular practice will help you glide farther and farther.

Don't sweat the small stuff—I've included a general guideline of how many steps to do with each part of the drill, but don't worry about getting an exact number of steps. It's best to get into a flow with this drill and not worry about how many steps you are taking—especially on the glide.

Smooth transition—Each time you shift gears you are using the momentum of the current mode to start you into the next mode. Don't make a sudden and abrupt change, but strive for a smooth transition between modes.

Here's how it's done:

- Start by walking for 30 seconds. Walk gently as you would walk during a walk break.

- Ease into running with a shuffle for 8-10 steps. This helps you transition from walking into running after a walk break.

- Next, ease into a slow jog for 8-10 steps and then a regular, easy pace for about 15 steps.

- If you have aches and pains or have no time goals, start your glide.

- Over the next 30 steps, those with time goals and free of aches and pains should gradually increase the speed to a fast but not all-out pace (approximately 5K race pace). Before an MM or a speed workout, gradually get into the pace you plan to run for that day.

- Now it's time to glide, or coast. Allow yourself to gradually slow down to a shuffle and then a jog using momentum as long as you can. You can train yourself to do this seamlessly.

- Continue to ease yourself into a walk break. As you do this regularly the transition will become smoother and smoother.

- At first you may only glide for maybe 10-15 steps. As the months go by you will get up to 20, then 30 and beyond. You're gliding!

- Walk for about 30 seconds as you would during a walk break.

- Repeat. Be in the moment! Do 4-8 of these.

Learning a smooth transition between running and walking: As you do this drill every week, you will feel smoother at each mode of running. You'll also develop a smooth and natural transition between running and walking...and running again (and again).

There will be some weeks when you will glide longer than others—don't worry about this. By doing this drill regularly, you will find yourself coasting or gliding down the smallest of inclines, and even for 10-20 yards on the flat, on a regular basis. Gliding conserves energy, reduces soreness and fatigue, and helps you maintain a faster pace in races with less effort.

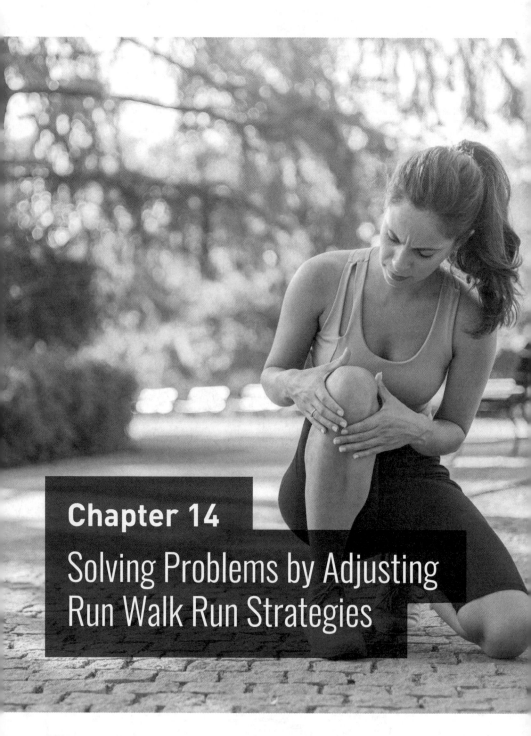

THE **RUN WALK RUN**® METHOD

Chapter 14
Solving Problems by Adjusting Run Walk Run Strategies

80

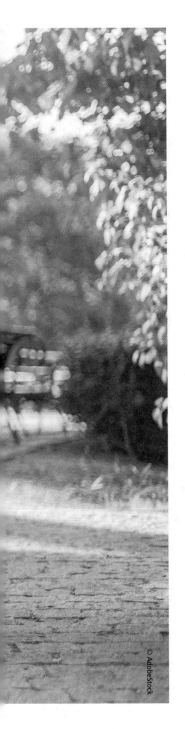

© AdobeStock

The **Run Walk Run** method is as close to a panacea for running problems as I've found during my more than half a century of running. By adjusting the amounts of running and walking, the body can recover better, adapt, erase fatigue, and avoid injury. This allows one to run farther, reduce or eliminate aches and pains, continue running while letting an injury heal, cope with heat, etc.

You are the captain of your running ship. By taking cognitive control over problems and setting up a strategy, you shift mental action into the conscious brain and away from the subconscious, emotional brain. As you adjust the Run Walk Run strategies you further empower the executive brain to evaluate, adjust, and come up with the right balance for that moment. The human, conscious brain activity will override the subconscious brain, allowing you to stay positive and focused. You can then manage the stress level, and reduce or eliminate the production of negative attitude hormones associated with running.

Don't get stuck in a rut. Run Walk Run adjustments can solve many problems and manage many more. But you must take action as soon as possible and continuously make adjustments as they are needed.

You first reaction should be to reduce your running significantly. The most common reason why runners hit a wall with fatigue, injury, etc. is that they don't cut back enough at first.

1. Aches and pains due to stress

Many runners experience more pains when under life stress or during the week or two leading to a tough goal race or other challenge. Many of these aches are due to a condition called Tension Myositis Syndrome (TMS) in which the overall stress level monitored by the subconscious brain stimulates it to constrict blood flow to certain areas that are already slightly damaged.

By taking executive mental action and adjusting walk break and goal focus, the subconscious reflex brain is no longer in charge, and blood flow resumes to the areas. Instead of not running, do a small amount of running with more walking—but get in your exercise. At the very least, walk for the amount of time or distance you would normally run. Exercise promotes blood flow. Many have reduced or stopped the pain during a 30-minute workout by mostly walking and visualizing the blood flow increasing to the area of pain.

Example: It's a very stressful week at work or you have a stressful meeting, exam, race, workout, etc. that is coming up. You have been running for 30 minutes, three times a week using a ratio of R3min/W1min. With no warning (or known cause), pain is noticed in an area that has not hurt previously or has only been a minor irritation.

Action: In most of these cases that I have monitored, there has not been a significant medical issue and there is no irritation of the problem when walking. Always consult a doctor if you suspect a real injury that could get worse by any running. Otherwise, write down your objectives in dealing with this. Suggested items are the following:

1. To get in a light exercise session to main adaptations

2. To stay below the threshold of further irritation during exercise

3. To run _____ seconds or minutes and walk _____ seconds or minutes

4. To mentally visualize the blood flowing to areas where there is irritation

5. To stop or walk gently if there is a significant increase in symptoms

6. To be confident that the pain will go away

The first action is to walk with a gentle stride for 5-10 minutes. If all is well, continue the gentle walk for the full length of a normal run. Usually this works without incident. Take a day off of running and do the next workout:

• Walk gently for 10 minutes

• Then R5-10 sec/W50-55sec. If there is no problem repeat for 4 minutes.

• If there are still no problems, move up to R10-15sec/W45-50sec.

• Do this for the rest of the workout if there are no problems.

• Have fun and be playful!

By continuing to exercise with a plan for each day, most of my runners with TMS have returned to regular running within two weeks—or less.

Note: Not all pains of this nature are due to TMS. For medical issues you should see a doctor. Try to find one who knows about TMS and wants you to run as you are able.

For more information on TMS and running, see my book *Mental Training for Runners*. The best source on TMS itself is *Mind-Body Prescription* by John Sarno, MD.

2. Running while injured

At some point, most runners experience some aches, pains, or injuries. With the right adjustment of less running and more walking, a high percentage of these issues (even significant ones) have gone away with little or no time off from running. The magic formula is to reduce the running amount and increase the walking.

The human organism is wired to heal itself if you let the process take place. I've worked with hundreds of injured runners, however, who had a big race on their calendar and kept pushing through the aches and pains until suddenly...breakdown. I believe that most would have prevented injury if they had backed off and used the right Run Walk Run strategy.

The good news is that most were able to run their race by using the method. At first, some time off of running was often required—only 3-5 days for most. Once the healing had started, either walking or running in short segments began.

Principle: Stay below the threshold of irritation. By reducing the amount of running enough, most of those who have come to me injured have been able to continue running while allowing the weak link to heal. Many have stayed on track toward their marathon or half-marathon goal.

Action: First determine whether or not walking for several miles will aggravate the injury. In most of the cases that I have monitored, walking is allowed. If not, find an alternative exercise (such as aqua-jogging or the ElliptiGO bicycle) that can maintain fitness without further irritation. Be sure there is not a significant medical issue that walking could aggravate. Always consult a doctor if you suspect a real injury that could be made worse by running. Be sure to tell the doctor that you will be running in very short segments at first (only 5-15 seconds every minute).

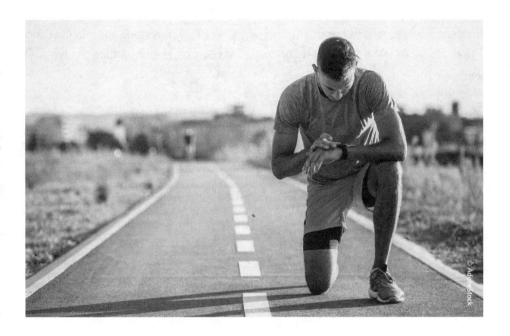

Next, write down your objectives in dealing with the injury. Suggested items are the following:

1. To engage in light exercise to maintain adaptations

2. To stay below the threshold of further irritation during exercise

3. To run _____ seconds or minutes and walk _____ seconds or minutes

4. To mentally visualize the blood flowing to areas where there is irritation

5. To stop or walk gently if there is a significant increase in symptoms

6. To visualize the healing circuits turned on and working to capacity

7. To believe in the healing process

THE **RUN WALK RUN**® METHOD

The first action is to walk with a gentle stride for 5-10 minutes. If all is well, continue the gentle walk for the full length of a normal run. Usually this works without incident. The next day you could do an alternative exercise such as aqua-jogging or ElliptiGO bicycle.

The next workout:

- Walk gently for 10 minutes

- Then R5-10sec/W50-55sec. If there is no problem repeat for 4 minutes.

- If there are still no problems, move up to R10-15sec/W45-50sec.

- Do this for the rest of the workout.

- Have fun and be playful!

- If you experience any problems, just walk.

- Walk or run with a short and gentle stride.

By continuing to exercise with a plan for each day, most of my runners with injuries have been able to complete their training schedule while allowing the injury to heal.

Note: This advice is given from one runner to another. For medical issues you should see a doctor. Find one who wants you to continue running.

No more injuries. All of us have weak links. These are the body parts that get irritated more often, resulting in aches, pains, and injuries. If you run continuously, you can expect to have the weak links talk to you at some point.

During my first 20 years of running I only took walk breaks on runs over 20 miles. During these two decades, I experienced a significant injury about every 20 days. Then, in 1978, I became a Run Walk Runner! For more than 35 years, I've not had a single running injury. I ran a marathon about every month for 15 years in my 60s and 70s using 15/15. I'm running marathon distance about once a month—more often than during my first 20 years!

There have been quite a few irritations of my weak links during the last three decades. In each case I did the following:

- Stopped running if there were significant injury symptoms

- Took 2-3 days off from running

- Applied treatment to the weak link if appropriate

- Tried a run with much more liberal use of walking

- Monitored weak link to stay below the threshold of irritation

- If there was irritation, walked gently for the rest of the workout

Significant Injury Symptoms

Inflammation—Swelling

Loss of function—The foot, knee, etc. doesn't function as normal

Pain—If pain is felt, and walking for 3-5 minutes does not help, STOP!

3. Run Walk Run adjustments to avoid injury

If you were using this ratio	Try this strategy
R3min or more/W1min or less	R30sec/W30sec
R1min/W1min or less	R15sec/W20-30 sec
R30sec/W30sec or less	R10sec/W30sec
R15sec/W30sec	R5-8sec/W30-40sec

If there is still some irritation when making one of the adjustments, walk for two workouts and come back with R5sec/W55sec. If this aggravates the injury, see a doctor. If not, then do the next workout at R5sec/W55sec for the first 10 minutes and then move up to R10sec/W50sec for 10 minutes.

Principle: Even small amounts of running will maintain most of the adaptations of running. But if you drop back to short enough run segments, the walking can usually stop the irritation. You're allowing the body to heal itself.

4. Coming back from an injury or illness

Most of the runners I've worked with who have experienced injury have been able to ease back into running after a few days off for healing. Illness presents more complex issues. Before resuming a strenuous training program after injury or illness make sure that your doctor has approved your return to running. The advice in this section and the book is from one runner to another. For medical advice, see a doctor.

By easing back into running using short segments, the legs, feet knees, etc. can gradually readapt naturally. Too much continuous running is the most common cause of injury. If walking is allowed during the time off from running, build the walk to 30 minutes. Whether walking or running, keep a short stride with your feet low to the ground.

Some runners will be able to progress more rapidly than others, but it is always best to start with very short segments of running. After about two weeks of very gentle running, most runners are able to add more running. Even then, a gradual increase back to the former level is recommended. Normally this is more than twice the time runners had to lay off from running due to injury, sickness, etc.

Principle: Stay below the threshold of further irritation of injury. When coming back from illness, be conservative in increasing workload. Too much, too soon can lower the immune system.

First run:

- Walk for the first 10 minutes.
- If all is well, move to R5sec/W55sec for 3 minutes.
- Walk for 3 minutes
- If all is well, gently try R5sec/W55sec for 4 minutes.
- Walk gently for 3 minutes.
- If all is well, gently try R5sec/W55sec for 5 minutes
- Walk gently for 10 minutes as a warm-down.

If there are no problems after the first workout, increase the number of R5sec/W55sec segments on successive workouts, every other day, until you're running 30 minutes. Don't do any strenuous exercise on the day off from running. Walking is usually allowed but ask your doctor.

Monitor weak links and back off if there is irritation.

Gradually increase the amount of running and decrease the amount of walking as the body adapts: R10sec/W50sec, R10sec/W40sec, R10sec/W30sec, R10sec/W20sec, R15sec/W30sec, R15sec/W30sec, R40sec/W30sec, R40sec/W20sec, etc.

If you feel that the irritation in an injured area is coming back, take 2-3 days off and come back with just a few minutes of R5sec/W55sec.

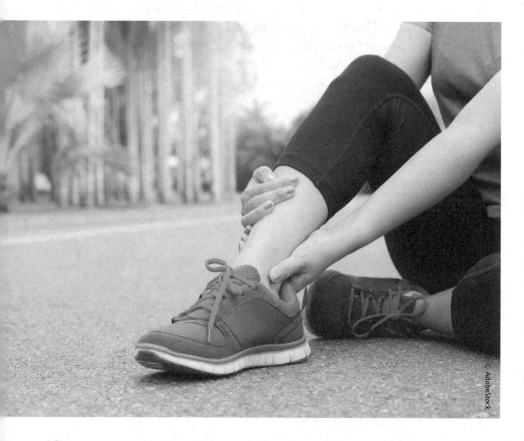

© AdobeStock

My comeback story: Returning to marathons after a hip fracture

By March 1, 2012, my wife Barbara and I had been running a marathon every month for about three years. I had just finished two days of filming a pilot for a TV show on running, and was walking up a stairway thinking about the next marathon in two weeks in Rome. As I reached the top of the stairwell, I noticed the doors opening ahead of me and shifted to the side, not looking at the top step. My left foot caught the lip, and my hip hit the stone floor hard, causing a fracture.

X-rays and an MRI disclosed three fractures. My excellent medical advisors, Dr. Ruth Parker and Dr. Paul Parker, believed that I should not jump into surgery or other procedures. I started learning how to use crutches. Barbara was so great about helping me get around. At first, almost any movement was awkward and any slight departure from a short range of motion triggered an instant jolt of pain.

Ruth told me right away that I should keep the calf muscle active and she suggested toe raises. I found that there was no pain doing these and I quickly built up to 700 per day. This was crucial in my return to running later.

I also walked around on crutches, several times a day. One day a week, I increased the distance covered on this long crutch run. This was simply a visualization—I imagined myself running along the sidewalk. Each week I went a bit farther.

Two weeks after the fracture I was scheduled to leave for Rome. My medical team was cautious but let me go. The RunItaly tour asked me to give clinics to the runners. I experienced a few moments of real pain trying to move from one mode of transportation to another and some significant swelling during and after the flights. But I crutched my way around Rome on the wonderful tours, and advised the runners on tour about how to be strong and energized during the marathon, while recovering fast enough to enjoy the tours and Italian cuisine. They seemed to believe me even if I was giving the clinics on crutches.

I continued my 700 toe raises each day for 7 weeks. During the sixth and seventh weeks, my bone seemed to be getting stronger every day, and I started supporting some of my weight on my legs when walking, while still getting some support from the crutches. Seven weeks after the day of the fracture, I felt strong enough to walk without crutches. I had many anxious moments that week. I walked around the house, up and down the hallways, then cautiously outside on the sidewalk. I was definitely wobbling as I walked through airports to my clinics. There was a lot of weakness due to the atrophy of the gluteus muscles, but the symptoms were not the pain I received from the bone damage. I talked this through with Ruth and Paul who cautioned me to monitor warnings as I increased the distance of my walk about every other day. The remaining damage seemed to be exclusively in the soft tissue in the gluteus medius and the many tendons, ligaments, nerves, and other components damaged during the fall.

During the two weeks of walking only, I increased my long walk distance to 8 miles. At that point, I felt that I could begin short running segments. I continued to feel weakness and significant soreness as I walked, but these symptoms seemed to lessen every two days or so. On my first attempt at running I was nervous and excited. I started with a 5-minute walk. Then I tried to jog for 5 seconds. I felt very awkward and unnatural, and walked for 55 seconds after each 5-second jog. On the first day, I did ten of these R5sec/W55sec segments and walked for 10 minutes. Every other day I increased the number of minutes of R5sec/W55sec until I could do 30 minutes.

Because of my toe raises, my calf muscles were ready to run. After 30 minutes of R5sec/W55sec, I moved up to R10sec/W50sec. The running felt more and more natural so I moved up to R15sec/W45sec and then to

R30sec/W30sec (one week at each ratio). At this point, I was at the Med City Marathon/Half Marathon in Rochester, MN, for clinics and decided to try the half marathon. While R30sec/W30sec felt doable at first, it was too much for the soft tissue when continuing for 13.1 miles. I shifted to R20sec/W20sec and finished with R15sec/W30sec walk.

I should have used R10sec/W20sec or R15sec/W30sec from the beginning. The extra stress of the R30sec/W30sec for that distance damaged the glute muscles, nerves, and tendons requiring a very gentle recovery week. I shifted back to R15sec/W30sec on my runs and started improving again. Two weeks later I used R15sec/W45sec to cover 15.5 miles. One month after Med City, I used R15sec/W45sec to cover 18 miles during the Grandma's Marathon, where I was giving advice about training and how to avoid tripping on stairwells.

There were no setbacks from the 18 miles, but soreness and glute weakness continued lessening every week. I planned to do 22 miles at the Missoula marathon, three weeks after Grandma's, and walk for the last 4 miles or so. It was a beautiful morning through the scenic Montana ranchland as I walked for 2 miles with my friends Kim and Stan. At that point, we decided to try R10sec/W20sec. It worked. At 22 miles I was having so much fun that I decided to continue and finished Missoula in 6:04. It was my slowest of 169 marathons but I couldn't have felt more proud or empowered.

For the first two days there was some of the usual glute soreness, but then it mostly disappeared. One month later I finished the Alaska Wild Life Marathon (one of my favorites) in 4:55 using R20sec/W20sec for the first half and then R15sec/W10sec for the second half.

The human body has an amazing ability to regenerate when challenged—if we let it.

5. Heat

Running will trigger a temperature increase. If the outside temperature is below 55°F, much of the body heat increase can be absorbed. But when running in temperatures of 65°F, 70°F, and above, core body temperature will continue to rise. Too much of an increase can result in a serious condition called heat disease which includes heat exhaustion and heat stroke.

Liberal walk breaks, from the beginning of a hot run, can minimize the internal heat increase. It's always better to err on the safe side of heat issues. Frequent walk breaks can not only keep you from overheating, you'll recover faster and finish stronger in races on warm or hot days.

On training runs, it's always better during hot weather to run in the pre-dawn hours, before the sun gets above the horizon. Shade will also reduce some of the heat stress generated by sunshine.

Remember: It's the length of the running segments that elevate core body temperature. By shortening the running segments and lengthening the walking segments, most runners can manage heat buildup on a hot day.

Note: If you suspect that you are in the preliminary stages of heat disease, cool off. Taking a cool shower for 5 minutes every 20-30 minutes of running, or walking gently for 10 minutes in an air-conditioned room every half hour can stop the temperature increase. If you experience extreme heat sensation, hot and cold flashes, cessation of sweating, extreme nausea, vomiting, or diarrhea, stop the workout and get help in cooling off immediately.

Here are recommended walk-break adjustments based upon temperature increase.

Run Walk Run Strategy Adjustments
With Temperature Increase

Starting pace/mi	< 55 °F	65 °F	70 °F	75 °F	80 °F	85 °F
9 min	R2min/ W30sec	R1:45min/ W30sec	R90sec/ W30sec	R80sec/ W30sec	R70sec/ W30sec	R60sec/ W30sec
10 min	R90sec/ W30sec	R80sec/ W30sec	R70sec/ W30sec	R60sec/ W30sec	R45sec/ W30sec	R30sec/ W30sec
11-12 min	R60sec/ W30sec	R50sec/ W30sec	R40sec/ W30sec	R30sec/ W30sec	R20sec/ W20sec	R15sec/ W20sec
13-14 min	R30sec/ W30sec	R25sec/ W30sec	R20sec/ W30sec	R15sec/ W20sec	R15sec/ W25sec	R15sec/ W30sec
15-16 min	R15sec/ W30sec	R10sec/ W30sec	R7sec/ W30sec	R5sec/ W30sec	Walk	Walk

Note: It is always appropriate to walk more and run less on a hot day to prevent heat disease.

Note: Be sure to slow down 30 sec/mi for every 5°F temperature increase above 60°F.

6. Hills

The right Run Walk Run strategy can take the sting out of almost any hill. By adjusting the running and walking portions according to the grade and the length of the hill, you can feel as strong at the top as you did at the beginning.

Take more frequent walk breaks! The calf muscle provides the prime propulsion up a hill. If you run continuously, that muscle will fatigue more rapidly. With more frequent walk breaks, the muscle can stay strong and resilient.

Personal records on the hilly Big Sur course

For many years I have given the training/racing clinics, the day before the beautiful Big Sur Marathon in Carmel, CA. The vistas on this course are spectacular, and are "earned" by going up and down the many hills. Non-stop runners who have compared times with average courses find themselves running about 20 minutes slower at Big Sur. Those who use the right Run Walk Run strategy have a different experience.

During these clinics I receive questions from many concerned runners who live in flat terrain areas like Chicago, New Orleans, Houston, etc. Having heard from thousands who have had great races on this course, I assure each that by using more frequent walk breaks on all uphills, the legs will be more strong and resilient during the wonderful downhills on that course. I have heard from dozens of the flat-landers who have run their fastest marathon on the Big Sur course because they took the advice.

Principle: Walking more frequently on the uphill sections saves energy resources and crucial muscle capacity for the last third of the race. Instead of slowing down and walking a lot at the end, those with the right Run Walk Run adjustments are strong to the finish. They are the passers not the passees during the last few miles which is very empowering.

Walking more on the uphill and using correct downhill form can allow you to eliminate some of the walk breaks on the downhills. Keep your feet low to the ground, use a relatively short stride, and let the ankles do most of the work. Through practice, most of my runners have been able to run quite fast without pounding the legs.

Run Walk Run Adjustments on Hills

Pace/ratio used on flat terrain	Pace/ratio used on average hill	Pace/ratio used on steep or long hill
9min/mi (R2min/W30sec)	9min/mi (R2min/W30sec)	R60sec/W30sec or R40sec/W20sec or R30sec/W30sec
10 min/mi (R90sec/W30sec)	10:15 min/mi using 60/30	10:30 min/mi using 40/25 or 40/30
11-12 min/mi using 60/30	11:20-12:20 min/mi using 40/20	11:40-13 min/mi using 40/25 or 30/30
13-14 min/mi using 30/30	13:20-14:30 min/mi using 25/30 or 20/25	13:40-15 min/mi using 20/20 or 15/30
15-16 min/mi using 15/30 or 10/30	15:30-16:30 using 10/30 or 10/40	16-17 min/mi using 10/30 or 7/23

7. Getting back on schedule

Almost every day one or more runners contact me because life got in the way of their training. Due to work, vacation, sickness, injury, or even all of the above, he or she missed several weeks of training or did not do the all-important long runs during a to-finish training program.

My message is one of hope. Thousands have reported their marathon or half-marathon success after following my advice to take more frequent walk breaks. By walking a lot more and running a lot less, the running body parts can readapt to the running motion without getting overwhelmed.

Principles:

1. Whether walking or running, it is the distance covered during the long run that determines the current endurance limit.

2. Even walking with no running will bestow all of the endurance, based upon the length of the walk.

3. When one has been away from running for an extended period (3 weeks or more), walking only should be used at first to rebuild the endurance. Gradually increase the duration of the walk to 30 minutes over the course of 2-3 weeks.

4. When it's time to start running again, gradually insert short jogging segments into the 30-minute walks every other day. Start with 5 seconds of jogging every minute. Then go to 10 seconds, then 15—over 2-3 weeks. Use one minute as the unit and subtract from the walking segment as you increase running. Find a ratio of running to walking that feels good to you—you don't have to shoot for running non-stop.

5. Allow the legs, feet, etc. to adapt. It's better to be conservative during the comeback.

6. If one mostly walks during the long weekend workouts to catch up with a race schedule, the same liberal walk strategy should be used in the race itself for at least the first half.

Catch-up training schedule

This assumes that there are no injuries and that you have been doing daily walking during the time off from running.

The example is a person who was on track for a half marathon but missed 4 weeks of regular running, including the 7-mile and the 8.5-mile long runs. This person had run a fastest MM of 9 minutes, and was running the long runs at 13:30 min/mi, using R30sec/W30sec. Runs on Tuesdays and Thursdays were 30 minutes long, using R60sec/W30sec, R90sec/W30sec, R60sec/W20sec and R3min/W1min.

Week	Long Workout	Tues/Thurs Workouts
1	3-5 mi walk	15-30 min each with 10 min of RWR
2	4-7 mi walk	20-30 min each with 15 min of RWR
3	5-9 mi walk	25-30 min each with 20 min of RWR
4	6-11 mi walk (2 mi RWR)	30 min each with 25 min of RWR
5	3 miles RWR	30 min each with 25 min of RWR
6	7-13 mi walk (4mi RWR)	30 min each with 25 min of RWR
7	3-4 miles RWR	30 min each with 25 min of RWR
8	8-15 mi walk (6 mi RWR)	30 min each with 25 min of RWR

Example:

Week	Long Workout	Tues/Thurs Workouts
1	3-5 mi walk	15 min: 5 min walk then 10 min of R10sec/W50sec
2	4-7 mi walk	20 min: W5min, then 15 min of R15sec/W45sec
3	5-9 mi walk	25 min: W5min, then 20 min of R20sec/W40sec
4	6-11mi–last 4 mi 15/45)	30 min: W5min, then 25 min of R35sec/W35sec
5	3 miles 20/40	30 min: W5min, then 25 min of R30sec/W30sec
6	7-13mi–last 6mi 15/45	30 min: W5min, then 25 min of R40sec/W20sec
7	3-4 miles (40/20)	30 min: W5min, then 25 min of R45sec/W15sec
8	8-15 mi–last 8mi 15/45	30 min: W5min, then 25 min of R60sec/W20sec

8. Heavier runners

Walk breaks have enabled thousands of very heavy sedentary citizens—some with joint problems—to become runners or return to running. Many have become marathoners. The use of very short run segments reduces the effort, the pounding, and the stress on weak links.

As noted in chapter 10, a gentle and gradual warm-up that includes short run inserts will allow most big bodies to adapt to the running motion. Some heavy runners don't run more than 10-20 seconds but experience the same joy, attitude boost, and vitality increase as others.

Each person must find their most gentle walking form. In general, a short stride with feet low to the ground reduces aggravations to the shins, feet, knees, etc. An upright posture tends to take stress off the back and the neck. Ease into the run, and glide into the walk.

Walk breaks are the shock absorbers to the system. At the first sign of huffing and puffing or aches to the weak links, insert more gentle walking and shorten the run segments. Many heavier runners who hit a fatigue wall during a run have walked gently for 5 minutes, reduced the running segments, and have finished the workout feeling better at the end.

Who is a heavy runner? Anyone who feels that their current body weight is making it more difficult to run can use the following Run Walk Run adjustments. Just pick the approximate number of pounds you feel you are overweight.

Pace per mile	10 pounds+	25 pounds+	40 pounds+	55 pounds+
9:00	R2min/ W30 sec	R1min/ W20sec	R40sec/ W15sec	R32sec/ W12sec
10:00	R90sec/ W30sec	R80sec/ W25sec	R60sec/ W25sec	R40sec/ W20sec
11:00	R80sec/ W45sec	R60sec/ W35sec	R50 sec/ W30sec	R30sec/ W20sec
12:00	R60sec/ W35sec	R40sec/ W25sec	R30sec/ W22sec	R20sec/ W20sec
13:00	R30sec/ W30sec	R20sec/ W20sec	R15sec/ W15sec	R10sec/ W15sec
14:00	R30sec/ W35sec	R20sec/ W25sec	R15sec/ W20sec	R10sec/ W20sec
15:00	R15sec/ W30sec	R12sec/ W22sec	R10sec/ W25sec	R10sec/ W30sec
16:00	R10sec/ W30sec	R8sec/ W30sec	R6sec/ W30sec	R5sec/ W30sec

Note: The Galloway Run Walk Run app is available from all app stores.

Note: On long runs, avoid huffing and puffing. If you start to breathe more heavily, drop back to more walking and less running.

9. Older runners

Walk breaks have enabled thousands of runners who were experiencing more aches and pains with passing years to get back into running. Many who had joint issues—including arthritis—have been able to continue running and often experience reduced symptoms. Using the right Run Walk Run strategy has allowed thousands to start running in their 60s and 70s.

Note: If you have medical issues, find a doctor who wants you to run and will help you do so if possible. For medical issues, ask a doctor.

Muscle capacity and performance decrease as we age. Unfortunately, many runners assume that they must give up running when they find it hard to run for a certain distance, such as a mile. The use of very short run segments has given older runners a new lease on their running life.

Research shows that runners have healthier joints than non-runners as the years go by. One study of runners over 50 who have been running for 20+ years showed that they experienced less than 25% of the orthopedic complaints compared with non-runners their age. Our bodies are designed to adapt to running and walking at any age and continue to benefit from these two activities as the years go by.

The most common reason why older runners retire from running is the increase in irritation of their weak links. Walk breaks allow the knees, hips, feet, etc. to gradually warm up and adapt to the running motion. Start with a gentle walk for 5 minutes. Then, insert 5-10 seconds of running into each minute of walking. Gradually increase the running time as the body warms up.

Walk breaks will reduce the effort of a workout, significantly reducing fatigue buildup. The Run Walk Run method can manage or eliminate the pounding and the stress on weak links, when the right strategy is used on a given day.

Older runners tend to run smarter because they have to solve more problems than younger ones. Each must find the most gentle and efficient form for running and walking, for the individual. In general, a short stride, with feet low to the ground has reduced aggravations to the shins, feet, knees, etc. An upright posture tends to take stress off the back and the neck. Ease into the run, and glide into the walk. Read the drills chapter in this book.

THE **RUN WALK RUN**® METHOD

Walk breaks are the shock absorbers to the system. At the first sign of huffing and puffing or aches to the weak links, insert more gentle walking and shorten the run segments. Many older runners who hit a fatigue wall during a run can turn this around by walking gently for 5 minutes, reducing the running segments, and adjust as needed.

Pace per mile	60+	70+	80+	90+
9:00	R2min/ W30 sec	R1min/ W15sec	R40sec/ W10sec	R32sec/ W8sec
10:00	R90sec/ W30sec	R60sec/ W20sec	R40sec/ W13sec	R30sec/ W10sec
11:00	R80sec/ W45sec	R60sec/ W35sec	R40 sec/ W25sec	R30sec/ W18sec
12:00	R60sec/ W30sec	R40sec/ W20sec	R30sec/ W15sec	R20sec/ W10sec
13:00	R30sec/ W30sec	R20sec/ W20sec	R15sec/ W15sec	R10sec/ W10sec
14:00	R25sec/ W30sec	R20sec/ W25sec	R15sec/ W18sec	R10sec/ W13sec
15:00	R20sec/ W40sec	R15sec/ W30sec	R12sec/ W24sec	R10sec/ W20sec
16:00	R10sec/ W30sec	R8sec/ W30sec	R6sec/ W30sec	R5sec/ W30sec

Note: The Galloway Run Walk Run app is available from all app stores.

Note: On long runs, avoid huffing and puffing. If you start to breathe more heavily, drop back to more walking and less running.

10. Walkers who want to go faster in races

By inserting short run segments into a walk, many walkers can pick up their pace and get to the finish line before officials shut it down. The gradual placement of run breaks will also allow the body to adapt to gentle running.

It is fine to walk exclusively during most of the long workouts leading to the race on the calendar. Many who have used this program, however, like to use 5-second run breaks every 2 minutes during the last 5-7 miles of the last 2-3 long workouts.

The long walks should be done every 2-3 weeks. On the alternate weekends, walk for 3-6 miles using the Run Walk Run strategy of choice, timing yourself on each mile to ensure that you can maintain closing pace for the race without huffing and puffing. As a reference, see *Galloway Training Programs* (visit *www.jeffgalloway.com*).

During the run segment, keep the feet low to the ground and touch lightly with the feet. Read the chapters in this book on running and walking form for more information.

One day a week, walk for 60 minutes. After a 10-minute walk, try various Run Walk Run segments such as the following:

Walk 55 seconds/run 5 seconds

Walk 50 seconds/run 10 seconds

Walk 25 seconds/run 5 seconds

Walk 30 seconds/run 7 seconds

Walk 25 seconds/run 4 seconds

Or choose the strategy of your choice.

11. Out of commission? Never again!

At some point, almost all runners have been exhausted after a long run. This is primarily due to too much continuous running—or simply not taking walk breaks often enough from the beginning. When the ratios are changed enough, most who run (even 26 miles) can carry on with normal family and friend activities after the run.

Heat can also be a cause of exhaustion. On hot days, strenuous workouts should be done before the sun rises above the horizon. Be sure to read and follow the instructions in the heat section of this chapter.

Rule #1: YOU CANNOT GO TOO SLOWLY OR TAKE WALK BREAKS TOO FREQUENTLY ON LONG RUNS.

Rule #2: When in doubt, walk slowly for several minutes and let the body restore itself.

Rule #3: Just walk the distance of the long run if you have serious challenges.

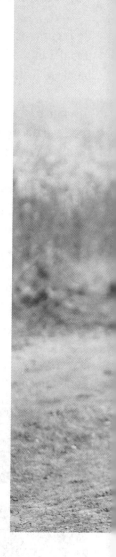

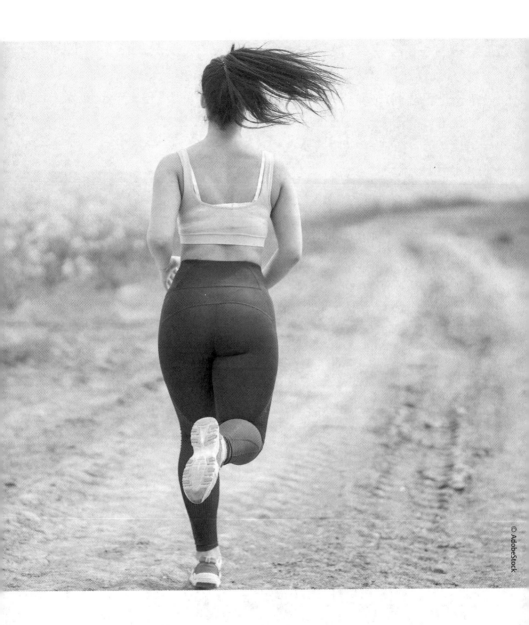

© AdobeStock

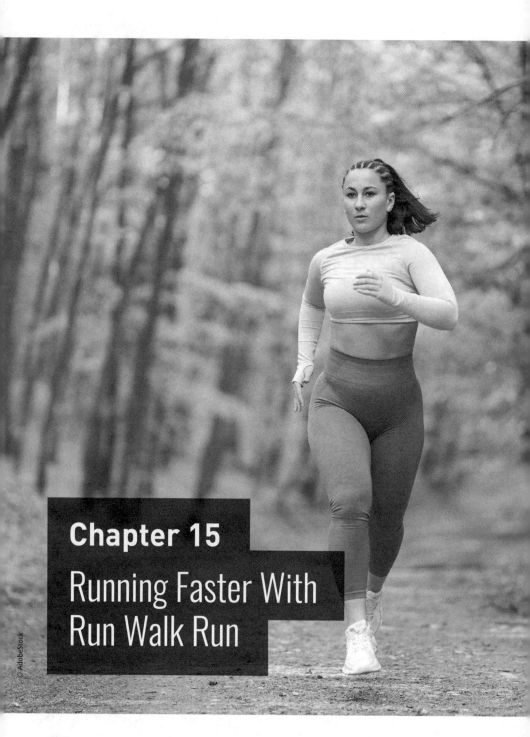

© AdobeStock

Chapter 15
Running Faster With Run Walk Run

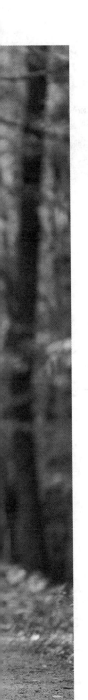

13 minutes faster: The average marathon improvement when non-stop runners shift to Run Walk Run.

7 minutes faster: The average half marathon improvement when non-stop runners shift to Run Walk Run.

Over 150 runners have reported a sub 3-hour marathon (6:52/mile pace) by using Run Walk Run—most could not run this fast when running continuously.

The fastest marathon time using Run Walk Run from the beginning is 2:28.

Many runners in the 12- to 16-minute pace range have reported running 60+ minutes faster in the marathon or 30+ minutes faster in the half marathon when they switched to Run Walk Run.

Over the past 40+ years I've received thousands of reports from former non-stop runners who improved finish times in a wide spectrum of race distances using my method. Even in the Magic Mile, over 80% of those who tried both running continuously and some form of Run Walk Run report a faster time by inserting some form of a walk break.

In longer distances, such as half or full marathons, those who run continuously almost always slow down significantly during the last third of the event. Those who use the right Run Walk Run strategy tend to maintain pace and in many cases speed up during the last 4 miles. In either case, the Run Walk Run folks receive a huge psychological boost as they pass person after person to the finish.

Principles:

Walk breaks must be taken from the beginning
Walk breaks must be used consistently
Walk breaks can be eliminated during the last third of the race, if desired

Boston qualified on a Run Walk Run bet

Jason had been running for about two decades, and encouraged his wife to join a Galloway program to start running. The Run Walk Run method allowed her to ease into running while meeting a great group of new friends. When she heard stories of faster running times by using the method she told Jason, but he knew that it wouldn't work for him—he had qualified and run in the Boston Marathon several times.

After failing to qualify for Boston three years in a row, Jason stepped up his training to run 3:10 or better—the time needed for his age group. He was on track for 17 miles and then painfully felt his pace get slower and slower, finishing in 3:23. Sensing that the method would avoid the slowdown at the end, Chris struck a deal. She wrote the family checks and he wanted a certain electronic product.

She said that if he would simply try using Run Walk Run in his next marathon, as written in *Galloway Training Programs*, she would buy him the equipment, but if he qualified he had to get up in front of the group and give his testimonial.

The day before his attempt, Jason came up to me, saying he wanted to clarify some points from my book. After asking him some questions about his pacing in several races I suggested a R6min/W1min strategy. I could tell that he was skeptical. A few weeks went by before I heard the outcome. Chris notified me that Jason had qualified and would tell the story before one of my upcoming clinics.

He explained to the group how Chris had offered the bet. He did the same training he had been doing for a few years but did not believe in the Run Walk Run method. This marathon had one purpose only—to win his bet with Chris.

The first 18 miles were right on pace as before, but this time he used R6min/W1min. He said that this mental strategy was just the opposite of the placebo effect—he knew he was going to fail. At mile 20, he was surprised that he was still on pace for his goal. By mile 23, he was tired but still strong and ran in to finish at 3:09.

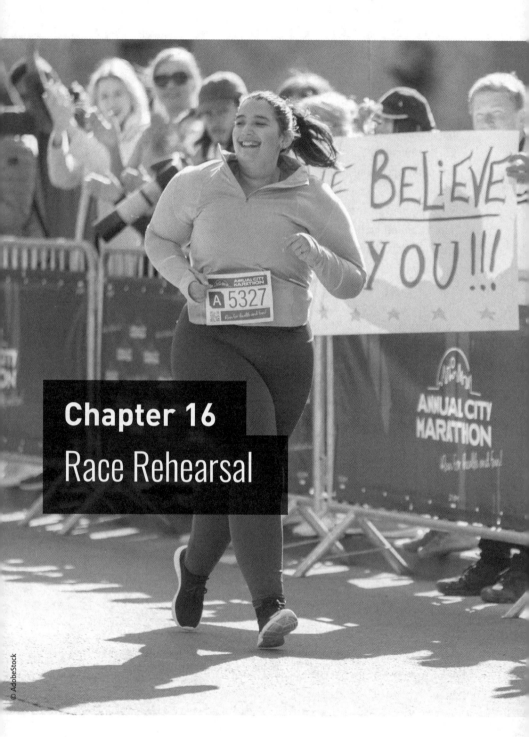

Chapter 16
Race Rehearsal

© AdobeStock

Practicing and choosing the right Run Walk Run strategy

The race rehearsal workout can help you experience goal race pace while testing several Run Walk Run strategies. By trying a variety of these strategies you will learn which feels best while having alternative strategies that you have used in case a shift is needed on race day. These workouts are scheduled on a short run day during each week—usually Tuesday or Thursday.

Magic Mile must predict goal pace

Before choosing a goal, look over chapter 7, especially the Galloway performance predictor in this book or at www.JeffGalloway.com. Make sure that your goal is in line with what is realistic.

Here's how to do the race rehearsal

After your warm-up, during one of the short runs each week, time yourself on a measured half-mile segment. Your mission is to run the time you want to run per half mile in the race.

For example, if your goal is 10 minutes/mile in the race, run the half mile in 5:00. Walk for 2-3 minutes between each. Repeat for 4-8 times. On each successive half mile (2 laps around a track) use a different Run Walk Run strategy. Here are some suggested alternatives based upon pace per mile.

Suggested pace strategies for race rehearsal segments

RACE REHEARSAL SEGMENTS
   8 min/mi
   - Run 4 min with a 30-second walk at the half
   - R2min/W15sec
   - R3min/W22sec

9 min/mi
- R2min/W30sec
- R80sec/W20sec
- R90 sec/W25sec

10 min/mi
- R90sec/W30sec
- R60sec/W20sec
- R45sec/W15sec
- R60sec/W25sec

11 min/mi
- R60sec/W30sec
- R50sec/W25sec
- R40sec/W20sec

12 min/mi
- R60sec/W30sec
- R40sec/W20sec
- R30sec/W20sec

13 min/mi
- R30sec/W30sec
- R20sec/W20sec
- R15sec/W15sec

14 min/mi
- R30sec/W30sec
- R30sec/W35sec
- R20sec/W20sec
- R20sec/W25sec
- R15sec/W15sec
- R15sec/W20sec

15 min/mi
- R15sec/W30sec
- R15sec/W35sec
- R10sec/W20sec
- R10sec/W25sec

16 min/mi
- R10sec/W30sec
- R8sec/W30sec
- R7sec/W30sec
- R6sec/W25sec

You want to feel smooth as you go through the half miles (800 meters). You'll learn how to pace yourself while experiencing which of the strategies feel smoother and which may allow you to stay on pace without significant effort.

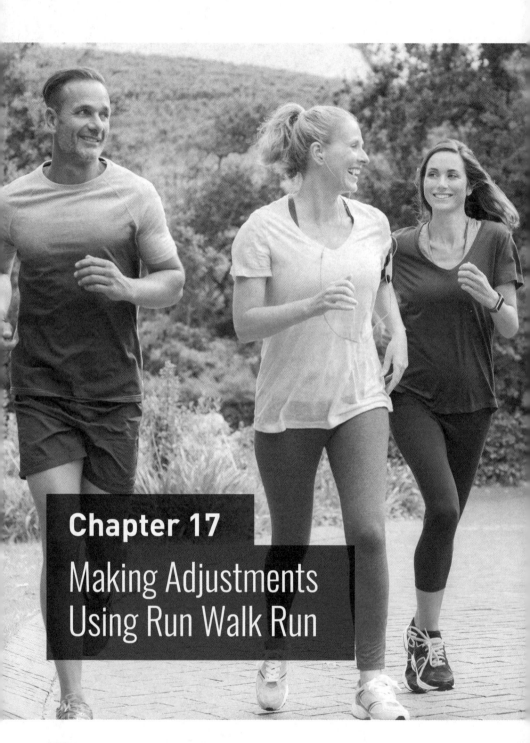

Chapter 17

Making Adjustments Using Run Walk Run

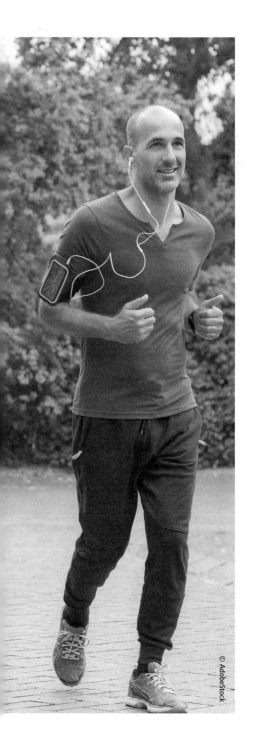

© AdobeStock

One of my favorite roles is helping runners solve problems. Almost every day I hear from at least one person who has experienced a rebirth of their running joy due to the Run Walk Run method. But I also work with runners who get stuck in a rut. Most commonly, a simple reduction in the running segment leaves the legs feeling stronger and recovering faster, while running faster in races. With more endorphins during a run, life is good—and running is better.

Over 35 minutes faster by dropping from R3min/W1min to R30sec/W30sec

Kathy signed on as an e-coach client with a best marathon time of 5:15. She was using a Run Walk Run ratio of R3min/W1min and was cramping during the last 5-6 miles. I asked her to try R1min/W1min and she improved by about 13 minutes. Because she still had some cramping issues I suggested R30sec/W30sec and she continued to improve down to 4:38.

Over an hour faster by changing from R3min/W1min to R20sec/W40sec

Cory weighed over 200 pounds with a marathon best of 6:15. He was slowing down a lot at the end of his marathons when using R3min/W1min. During his first marathon at R1min/W1min, he broke 6 hours! But there were a few cramping episodes during the last few miles so I asked him to try R30sec/W30sec. He liked this and continued to improve to 5:50. One month before his current time goal marathon, Cory entered a marathon as a training run. In efforts to keep him from running too fast I asked him to do the long-run marathon using a strategy of R20sec/W40sec. When he sent me his weekly e-coach report he was proud to say that he followed my advice but that it hadn't turned out as planned.

When only running for 20 seconds, Cory found he could run much faster because he had 40 seconds of walking for recovery. His finish time was 5:20—a 30-minute personal record. During the next year, he used a combination of R20sec/W40sec and R30sec/W30sec to improve down to 5:05.

Rules of adjustments

1. Never hesitate to drop back to more walking and less running.

2. Take a longer walk break if a challenge is approaching (e.g., hill, heat, pain).

3. If things aren't going well at the beginning of a workout or race, ease back and walk more. Often the body will rebound with strength later.

4. When facing one of the challenges below at the end of a workout and if you are exhausted—and not injured or sick—walk the rest of the distance.

5. If things are not going well in a race, revert to training pace with the Run Walk Run strategy used on long runs and you can race again in 3-4 weeks.

6. Read the section on solving problems for details about Run Walk Run strategies that have worked for various situations.

The standard Run Walk Run strategies mentioned in this book have worked well for thousands of runners who have overcome each challenge mentioned. But each of us has individual issues, and will commonly have different body and mind responses at different times of the year.

Be sure to read chapter 14 on solving problems for specific strategies on these challenges:

- **Aches, pains, and injuries**—The insertion of liberal walk breaks can often allow runners to keep training while the injured area heals.

- **Slowdown at the end of long runs and races**—The insertion of more frequent walk breaks from the beginning will keep the legs strong to the end. Practice several strategies during your race rehearsal segments.

- **Heat issues, body shuts down.** On hot days, much more walking allows runners with low heat tolerance to finish long runs and stay on track for the goal.

- **Feeling out of commission after long runs**—No need to experience this if you use the correct Run Walk Run strategy from the beginning: shorten the run segments and increase the walks.

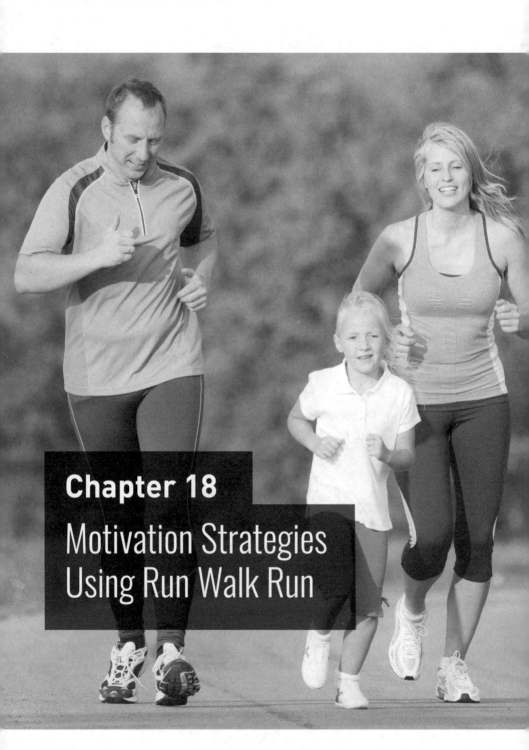

Chapter 18

Motivation Strategies Using Run Walk Run

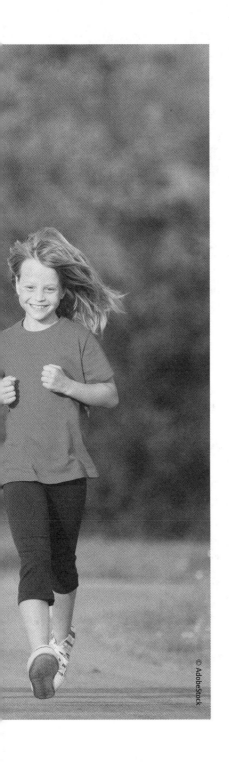

© AdobeStock

Finishing a tough workout or race

You're into a hard workout, your times are slowing down and you feel really tired. By focusing on the negative thoughts, you'll increase overall stress and allow the subconscious brain to trigger negative attitude peptides, injecting billions of cells with their low motivation messages. If you don't have a cognitive strategy, you'll find yourself thinking thoughts such as:

- This isn't your day.

- You can't reach your goal today.

- Just slow down a little.

- There are other days to work hard.

- Do this workout again when you are more motivated.

Evaluate whether there is a real reason (e.g., medical, heat, etc.) why you can't run as projected. If there is a reason, back off and conserve—there will be another day.

Almost every time, however, the problem is more simple: you are not willing to push through the discomfort. You are allowing the subconscious brain to stimulate negative attitude hormones, reducing your desire to do your best.

121

The most effective way to turn attitude around is to change the ratio of the Run Walk Run strategy you are using.

Mentally focus on the next segment of the workout. If you have been using R3min/W1min and were slowing down during the last minute, reset to R60sec/W30sec. As you find a segment of running that you know you can do, you gain confidence and release positive hormones. More positive secretions push your mood to the positive and keep the negative emotions away.

Reset your timer if needed. Taking the positive action of evaluating the segments on your Run Walk Run timer will shift control into the frontal lobe of your brain and into the executive center. You will set a strategy that works so that you feel confident that you can run for the number of seconds or minutes in your running segment. If you have any doubt that you can run for that period, then reset to a shorter amount.

Focus only on the next running segment.

Say positive things like "I'm pushing back my barriers," "I'm overcoming challenges," and "This is making me tougher." As you add to the number of repetitions during each workout and talk to the frontal lobe, you allow it to reprogram the reflex brain and lock into a series of steps to get through the fatigue at the end of the workout. By the time you run the goal race, the reflex brain is ready to click into one positive step at a time to get to the end.

Confront the subconscious brain's negative messages with strength statements like

"Don't quit!" "I can run one more minute," "I can run 30 more seconds," and "I can run 15 seconds!" Mental toughness starts with simply not giving up. Ignore the negative messages, stay focused on the next few steps, and talk to yourself. Focusing on a doable length of run segments shifts control to the executive brain and away from the reflex brain. Positive affirmations activate positive peptides.

I can do the next segment! By focusing on the next running segment, and shortening the length if needed, you are in cognitive control over your run.

In your speed workouts, practice the following drill. Fine-tune this so that when you run your goal race, you will have a strategy for staying mentally tough, with a flood of positive peptides.

The scene:
You're getting very tired, you'd really like to call it quits, or at least slow down significantly.

Quick strategies
Break up the remaining workout into segments that you know you can do:

- Tell yourself "Just one more minute." Run for one minute, then reduce pace slightly for a few seconds. Then say "Just one more minute" again, and again. Other segments that have been successful are the following: 30 seconds, 20 seconds, and 10 seconds.

- Tell yourself "Just 10 more steps." Run about 10 steps, take a couple of easy steps, then say "Just 10 more steps."

- Tell yourself "One more step." Keep saying this over and over—you'll get there.

Take some gliding breaks
- Reduce the tension in your leg muscles and feet by gliding for a few strides every 1-2 minutes. The acceleration-glider drill prepares you for this moment, particularly when coasting downhill.

- As you say "I'm gliding" or "I'm running smoothly," you continue the mental shift to the positive.

Segment by segment

- If you really question your ability to get through the workout, start each repetition, or race segment, saying to your self—"just one more" (even if you have 4 to go) or "10 more steps". "I'm getting it done!"

- Teamwork! You may not realize it but you are on a team of thousands around the country and the world, who are using the Run Walk Run method. You can pull motivation from the other person or persons. Think about your team members and say to yourself: "I feel their strength." The perception of team bonding can pull you through many difficult workouts and shift your attitude hormones in your favor.

- When you are getting close to the end and really feel like you can't keep going, say to yourself "I am tough," "I can endure," "Yes, I can," or "One more step."

- Smile!

Finishing a tough race

At any stage of a hard race—even in the first third—you can encounter problems that bring doubt and trigger negative messages from the reflex brain. If you focus on these messages, you will produce negative attitude hormones that will lower your motivation.

- By rehearsing every negative message you could get, you will desensitize yourself to their attitude lowering effect.

- Confront each negative with a positive statement. Start with something you can control: the length of the run segment. Say to yourself: "I can walk in 60 seconds." If this is questionable, reduce it to 30 seconds, or 20, or 10. The race or the workout is simply a series of segments. Don't focus on the distance left in the race, just how long you will run before you walk.

IF YOU FEEL NEGATIVE...	MAKE A POSITIVE STATEMENT.
Back off, this isn't your day.	Don't give up!
Thirty-second segments are getting tough.	I will run for 20 seconds.
There are other races.	I can do it.
Why are you doing this?	I'm getting tougher.

- **Evaluate whether there is a real medical reason (which is rare). If there is a health problem, back off and conserve—there will be another day.**
  Most commonly, the subconscious reflex brain is responding to the stress buildup of the workout/race by triggering negative peptides, creating a negative emotional environment. A successful strategy during the first onset of this attitude downturn is to glide a little. If needed, take an extra walk break (2-3 minutes) to mentally re-group and focus on the next segment of the race.

- To do your best in a race, you must manage the stress buildup by using a routine such as those that follow. You are training yourself to keep going, which is 90% of the battle. You are also programming the conscious brain to regularly check on the reflex brain, stop the negative thoughts, and insert positive beliefs.

- Continue to confront monkey brain messages with strength statements: Don't quit! I can do it!

- In your speed workouts, practice the following drill. Fine-tune this so that when you run your goal race, you will have a strategy for staying mentally focused and positive. Your belief in a plan will increase the production of positive motivational hormones.

The scene: You're getting very tired and stressed in a race, you'd really like to call it quits, or at least slow down significantly.

Quick strategies

- Break up the remaining race into segments that you know you can do.

- Tell yourself "Just one more minute." Run for one minute, then reduce pace slightly for a few seconds, then say "One more minute" again, and again (or 30 seconds, or 15 seconds, etc.).

- Tell yourself you will take just "Ten more steps." Run about 10 steps, take a couple of easy steps, then say "Ten more steps."

- Tell yourself "One more step." Keep saying this over and over—you'll get there.

- Take an extra walk break to gather yourself if you need it.

- Take some gliding breaks. By doing the acceleration-glider drill, you will be prepared to do this in the race.

- Reduce the tension in your leg muscles and feet by gliding for a few strides every 1-2 minutes. The acceleration-glider drill prepares you for this moment, particularly when coasting downhill.

Segment by segment

- In the race, if you really question your ability to finish, start each race segment, saying to yourself—"just one more" or "10 more steps". You'll make it the whole way.

- Teamwork! You are needed by the team. Belonging to a larger group with team spirit can pull you through many difficult workouts. Even if you have a long-distance friend that you are going to report to, it helps to have that connection. Some runners bring their cellphone on long runs and call their friend as a lifeline, during the walk breaks.

- When you are getting close to the end and really feel like you can't keep going, say to yourself "I am tough," "I can endure," "Yes, I can," or "One more step."

"I CAN DO IT... I AM DOING IT... I DID IT!

Mantras

Mantras can distract you from negative feelings generated by the subconscious brain under stress. But they can also actually shift mental gears. When you say a mantra and think about the meaning of the words, you stimulate the conscious brain. This component can override the negative actions of the subconscious brain and allow you to stimulate positive attitude hormones.

Having a list of mantras that deal with Run Walk Run issues will keep you focused on the next run segment and then the next walk break. This is a cognitive strategy that keeps you in control over your attitude.

As you say each mantra over and over, believe in it. If you need to edit to believe, do it.

- **I'm in control!**
- **I can change the run amount.**
- **I can change the walk amount.**
- **I have the strength.**
- **On to the next walk break!**
- **I can run _____ (amount of the run segment).**
- **One run at a time.**
- **One walk at a time.**
- **Walk breaks erase fatigue.**
- **I can do it!**
- **Run Walk Run to the finish line.**

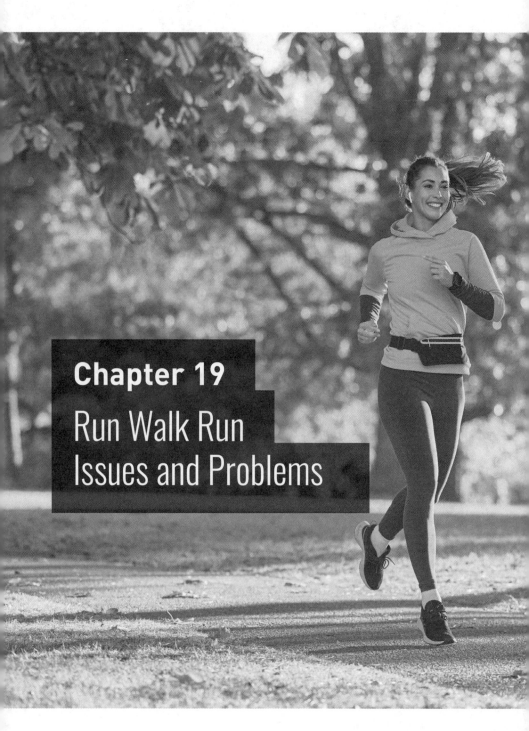

Chapter 19
Run Walk Run
Issues and Problems

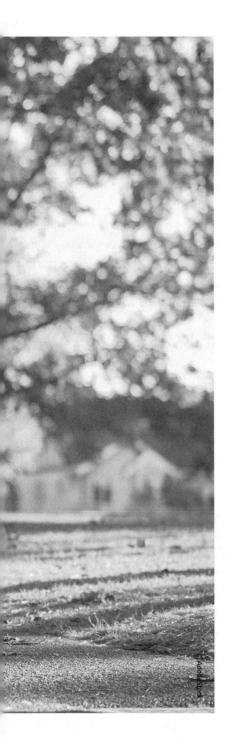

How fast do I have to run during my running segment to maintain a certain pace in a race?

Sorry, but I can't tell you. In numerous surveys we've found that runners run and walk at different paces during a long race or training run. To stay on pace, look at your stopwatch each mile. If you are too fast, take an extra walk break. If you are too slow, pick up your running pace during the next mile.

Knees, hips, or legs tighten or ache when going into a walk break or coming out of one.

Be sure to do the acceleration-glider drill which is described in chapter 13. By doing 4-8 of this AG every week, you can teach yourself to seamlessly move from a walk into a shuffle, easing then into a slow jog, a regular jog, and then gliding gently back into a walk. Practice makes you seamless.

It is hard to start up after a walk break.

Don't walk longer than 30 seconds, and work on the AG drill every week. Shortening the run segment has reduced fatigue at the end of runs. At the end of races, if you are having trouble getting back into the run, just shuffle through the walk breaks.

129

Slowing down at the end of a running segment.

This is usually due to having run segments that are too long. Try shortening both the run and the walk segments.

Walk breaks mess up my rhythm.

When runners start using the method or change to shorter segments, this is a common complaint. The primary benefit of the right Run Walk Run strategy is strong legs at the end of a race or long run, and quick recovery. The human organism is capable of adapting to changes in rhythm and timing the run and walk segments speeds up this process. There are wonderful benefits from making the shift: faster times, never being out of commission after a long run, and passing people at the end of a race. Practice can get you into a new rhythm, with all the Run Walk Run benefits.

My running friend doesn't want to take walk breaks.

Just ask your friend to try the method on one long run. In most cases the benefits are dramatic and you have a new convert. You can certainly run non-stop on short runs together. But if the friend chooses not to take walk breaks on long runs, explain that you need to stay injury free, avoid exhaustion, and enjoy friends and family after long runs—and Run Walk Run allows you to do this.

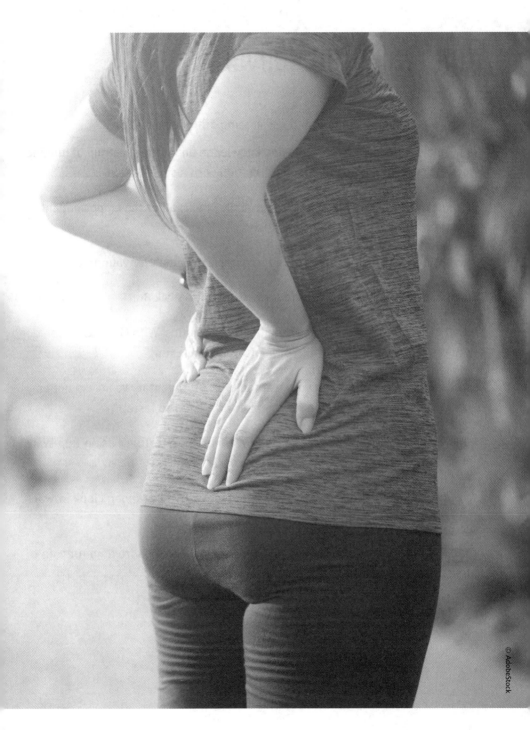

© AdobeStock

Run Walk Run delivers....

Faster races, no more injuries, and never being out of commission!

"Jeff Galloway not only has an amazing knowledge about the spectrum of running issues, he cuts through conflicting information with a simple plan."

"Run Walk Run is taking over because it really works: all of the empowerment of finishing with no more pain and exhaustion."

"There is no way I would have started running if it weren't for your method."

"I qualified for the Boston Marathon because of Run Walk Run."

"I used to be out of commission after all of my long runs. With Galloway, I can do anything with my family, friends—even after a 26-mile run!"

"I started running again using your method after 20 sedentary years. I'm not only experiencing the joy of running for the first time, I'm also faster!"

"A friend improved his best time for the 5K from 19:07 to 16:47 using Run Walk Run and won the race!"

"Your method of Run Walk Run has turned me into a HAPPY runner; I look forward to my training."

"Your program is amazing. PERIOD. I see men and women go from no running to half marathons regularly now."

"You delivered what you promised. You got me across the finish line smiling, and injury free."

"Everything you said was 100% right on. I was so strong at the finish it amazed me!"

"I felt the very best that I have ever felt after a full marathon. I was recovered and ready to run the following morning."

"Because of your method my love-hate relationship with running has turned into a love-love relationship. I've PR'd in my last two races and simply feel great!"

"Your training programs have gotten me to where I am today. I couldn't run one quarter mile, now I'm a Boston Qualifier. "

"Jeff, your methods and education have changed my life forever. In just one year I went from 44 years old and ZERO exercise for the past 20 years to 45 lbs. lighter and just ran a 4:41 marathon."

"Before your program I was not able to run to the end of my street. I have lost almost 70 lbs. since I met you earlier this year and have run 3 marathons."

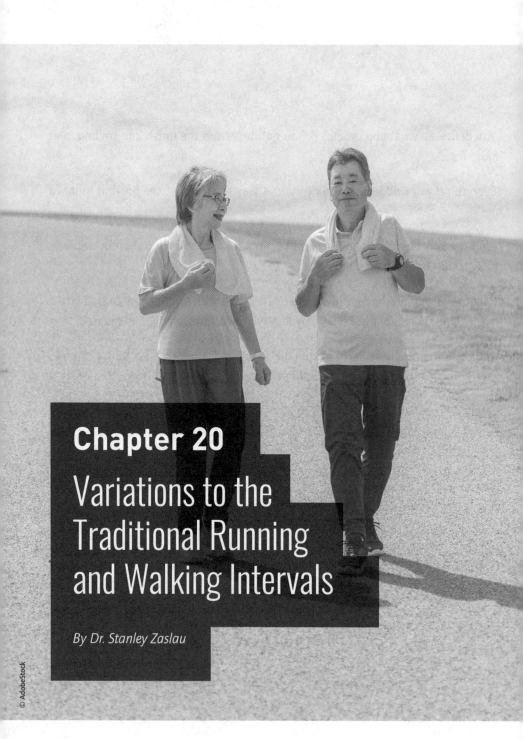

Chapter 20
Variations to the Traditional Running and Walking Intervals

By Dr. Stanley Zaslau

Here are the benefits I've received by continuing to adjust the running and the walking amounts:

- Improved leg turnover

- Development of a comfortable stride and running motion

- Better recovery during the walk interval

- Recovery from injury while staying below threshold of injury

- Ability to run faster with confidence

Athletes may find that variations to the traditional running and walking intervals may be beneficial in several settings:

- The beginning runner can gently introduce the body to running by using very brief periods such as 5 seconds. Thus, they could run for 5 seconds and walk for 55 seconds to allow some use of the running muscles followed by a long period of recovery.

- Short running intervals allow the injured Run Walk Run athlete to return to running while staying below the threshold for injury. The athlete can begin with running for 5 seconds followed by a walk for 55 seconds for the initial week back from injury. If things go well, they have several choices to make to improve speed. They can increase the running interval from 5 seconds to 10 seconds or they can reduce the walk break from 55 seconds to 45 or 50 seconds. This could create a new ratio for the next recovery week of R10sec/W50sec. If the body responds well, the interval can be further adjusted to R15sec/W45sec. If the muscles are not responding, the former ratio can be used.

SAMPLE INJURY RECOVERY PLAN	
Week	Run Walk Run Interval
1	R5sec/W55sec
2	R10sec/W50sec
3	R15sec/W45sec
4	R10sec/W40sec or R20sec/W40sec

- One can modify traditional Run Walk Run intervals to improve speed through improved leg turnover. For example, an athlete who uses R30sec/W30sec but tires towards the end of races can try intervals such as R20sec/W20sec or R15sec/W15sec with desired results in improvement in training or race time. Athletes are encouraged to try these intervals during their weekly training runs to see which ones work better for them. Further modification of traditional Run Walk Run intervals are also possible. Athletes have reported significantly improved times with intervals such as R10sec/W20sec.

- Even somewhat innovative intervals such as R12sec/W17sec, which is a variation of R25sec/W35sec, can produce faster times. How is this possible? With shorter running intervals, athletes can run these intervals with increased leg turnover and an increased stride length. For a brief time period, the athlete will become minimally fatigued and allow for the running muscles to recover during the walk break. Most runners will have their most significant improvement in fatigue during the first 10-15 seconds of the walk break so that the 20 seconds of walk in the R10sec/W20sec example can produce rather fast times overall. One could expect to maintain a pace of 13 minutes/mile or faster with practice.

Use of mathematics to create the best Run Walk Run interval based on traditional Galloway Run Walk Run intervals

Each athlete can create the Run Walk Run interval that works best. However, if you want to take the guesswork out of the formula, here is a thought. For the Run Walk Run interval of R20sec/W40sec, the ratio of running to walking is .50. If this is the ratio you want to use but you want to try a similar variation, one could try R10sec/W20sec, or R5sec/W10sec. While these are certainly short intervals, similar longer intervals can be created such as R40sec/W80sec, R1min/W2min depending on the fitness of the athlete. The choice is up to each athlete and the best way to figure this out is to try it out. Below are some samples of interval variations that have worked for some athletes that are nontraditional:

- R25sec/W35sec

- R10sec/W20sec

- R12sec/W17sec

- R15sec/W20sec

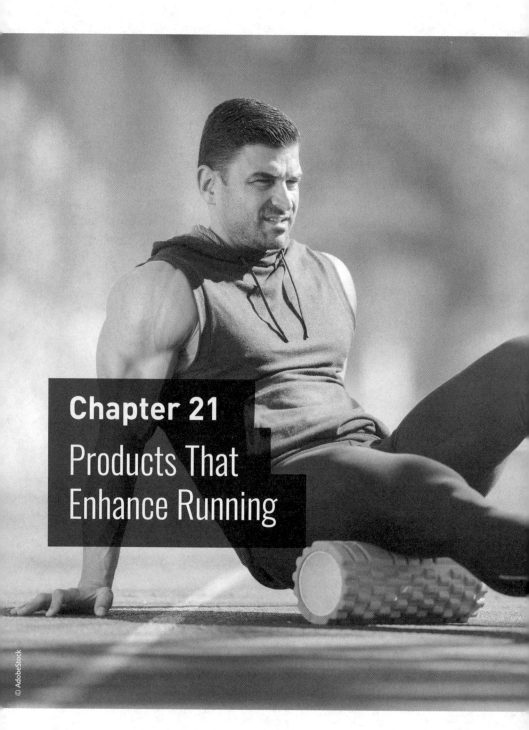

Chapter 21

Products That Enhance Running

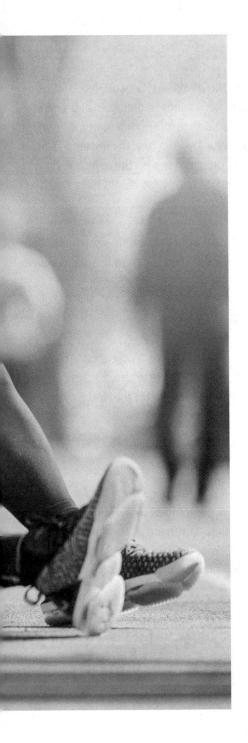

The stick

This massage tool can help the muscles recover faster. It will often speed up the recovery of muscle injuries or iliotibial band injuries (on the outside of the upper leg, between knee and hip). This type of device can help warm up the legs muscles and sore tendons before running, and move some of the waste out afterward.

In working on the calf muscle—most important muscle in running—start each stroke at the Achilles tendon and roll up the leg toward the knee. Gently roll back to the origin and repeat. For the first 5 minutes your gentle rolling will bring additional blood flow to the area. As you gradually increase the pressure on the calf you will usually find some knots or sore places in the muscles. Concentrate on these as you roll over them again and again, breaking up the tightness.

Foam roller

A foam roller can be used in self-massage for the iliotibial (IT) band, hip, and other muscles. The most popular size of this cylinder is 6 inches in diameter and one foot long. This has been the most successful treatment device for IT band injury. In treating this injury, put the roller on the floor, and lie on your side so that the irritated IT band area is on top of the roller. As your body weight presses down on the roller, roll up and down on the area of the leg you want to treat. Roll gently for 2-3 minutes and then let the body weight press down more.

This is a very effective pre-warm-up exercise for any area that needs more blood flow as you start. It is also very beneficial to use the roller after a run on the same areas.

The Jeff Galloway BFF Vibration Massager

This is the best instrument I have found for helping muscles to recover fast. According to experts, it helps to bring increased blood flow to the muscles for quicker recovery and repair. The muscles are invigorated and feel so much better the next day.

Accelerade

This sports drink has a patented formula shown to improve recovery. It also helps to improve hydration. I recommend having some in the refrigerator as your fluid intake product taken throughout the day. The prime time to drink this regularly is the day before and the day after a long or strenuous workout day. During a prolonged speed-training session, have a thermos nearby for sipping during walk breaks.

Research has also shown that drinking Accelerade about 30 minutes before running can get the body's start-up fuel (glycogen) activated more effectively, and may conserve the limited supply of this crucial fuel

Endurox R4

This product has what I see as a cult following among runners. Research shows that the 4:1 ratio of carbohydrate to protein helps to reload the muscle glycogen more quickly. This means that the muscles feel bouncy and ready to do what you can do sooner. There are other antioxidants that speed recovery. The prime time for this reloading process is within 30 minutes of the finish of a run.

Your Personal Running Journal

This is my training journal. It has week-by-week entries with graphs and instructions and can be ordered from *www.JeffGalloway.com*, autographed. It simplifies the process with places to fill in information for each day. Your journal allows you to organize your training in advance, which you can use as a daily workout guide. As you plan ahead and enter your data, you gain control over your training.

Other Galloway books, training schedules, and gifts that keep on giving

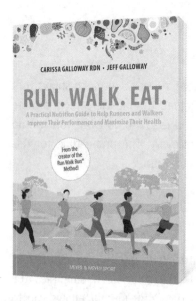

Run. Walk. Eat.
Coauthored with registered dietitian nutritionist (and my daughter-in-law) Carissa Galloway, this book gives all runners the best nutrition advice to eat to fuel their runs and to feel healthy.

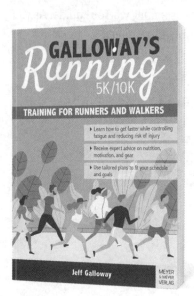

Galloway's 5k/10k Running
Whether you want to finish with a smile on your face or reach a challenging time goal, this book is a total resource for these distances. There are schedules for a wide range of performances; tips on how to eat, how to predict your performance, and how long and how fast to run on long runs; and drills to improve form and speed training. There is also extensive information on mental preparation, breaking through barriers, practical nutrition, and more.

Running Until You're 100

In the chapter on joint health, you'll see research studies showing that runners have healthier joints than sedentary folks. In the chapter on the researched health benefits of exercise, an expert on longevity says that for every hour we exercise we can expect to get back two hours of life extension. In the heroes section, you'll discover an 85-year-old man who recently finished his 700th marathon and will do 29 more this year. There are nutrition suggestions from Nancy Clark, training adjustments by decade, and many other helpful hints for running past the century mark.

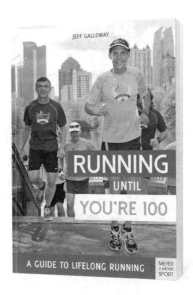

Mental Training for Runners

This has been a breakthrough resource for those who struggle with motivation issues in starting a workout, pushing through adversity, breaking through barriers at the end of a hard workout or race, and many more situations. You'll learn why we lose our motivation and what we can do to turn this around. There are training methods for maintaining control over attitude, drawing on past success, staying mentally focused, etc. The chapter on mantras covers a variety of challenges with positive thoughts and statements.

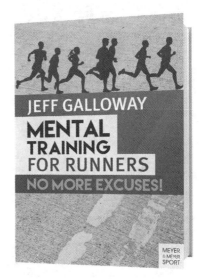

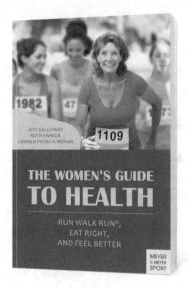

The Women's Guide to Health
This action guide combines the Run Walk Run program with the best available medical knowledge for using Run Walk Run and the Mediterranean Diet as key treatment modalities for chronic medical conditions related to excess body weight.

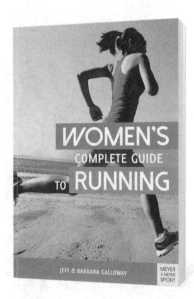

Women's Complete Guide to Running
by Barbara and Jeff Galloway
The section on woman-specific issues makes this book unique: pregnancy, menstrual issues, bra-fitting, incontinence, osteoporosis, inner organs shifting, menopause, and more. There's also a section for the unique problems of the fabulously full-figured runners. Nutrition, fat burning, motivation, starting up, and aches and pains are all covered in the book. There's also a section written by famous sports nutritionist Nancy Clark.

Half Marathon:
A Complete Guide for Women
by Barbara and Jeff Galloway
Women are flooding into half marathons as an empowerment experience. This book explains the process with schedules whether your goal is to improve your time or to cross the finish in the upright position. New to this book is a section on how to burn fat while training for a half marathon. There is also a section on women-specific issues

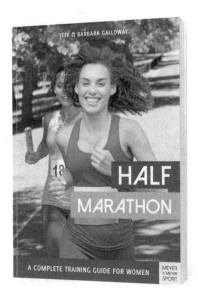

Running and Fat Burning for Women
by Barbara and Jeff Galloway
I've not seen another book that better describes the fat-burning and accumulation processes with a strategy to take action. There are several important and inexpensive tools mentioned, with recipes and specific suggestions about managing the calorie income and expenditure. There is also a section on women-specific issues. The principles of fat burning work for men also.

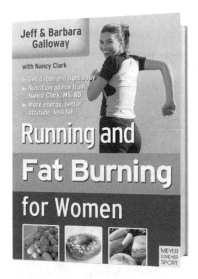

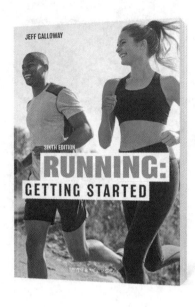

*Running –
Getting Started*
This is more than a state-of-the-art book for beginners. It gently takes walkers into running with a 6-month schedule that has been very successful. Also included is information on fat burning, nutrition, motivation, and body management. This is a great gift for your friends or relatives who can be infected positively by running.

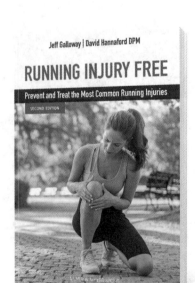

*Running Injury Free –
Prevent and Treat the Most
Common Running Injuries*
Dave Hannaford is one of the best resources I've found in explaining why we get injured and how we heal. He breaks down each major running injury to help you diagnose, treat, and heal. I have written the section on prevention based upon more than 30 years of no overuse injuries.

Galloway's Half Marathon Training
This new book provides highly successful and detailed training schedules for various time goals for this important event. Information is provided on nutrition, mental preparation, fluids, race-day logistics and checklist, and much more.

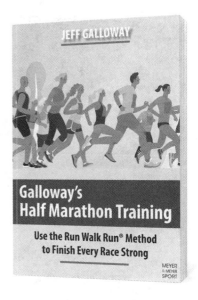

Galloway's Book On Running 2nd Edition
This is the best-seller among running books since 1984. Thoroughly revised and expanded in 2001, you'll find training programs for 5Ks, 10Ks, and half marathons with sections on nutrition, fat burning, walk breaks, motivation, injuries, shoes, and much more. This is a total resource book!.

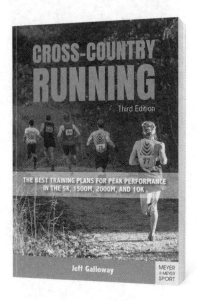

Cross-Country Running – Third Edition

Record numbers of young people are joining cross-country teams at the high school and junior high level. This book has pre-season and in-season training for the various cross-country events with nutrition, motivation, injury trouble-shooting, and other backup information. Specific chapters are included on strategy, hill training and technique, running form, efficiency drills, terrain training, and much more.

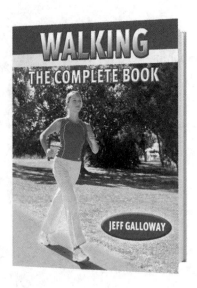

Walking:
The Complete Book

Walkers now have a book that explains the many benefits of walking and how to maximize them with training programs for 5Ks, 10Ks, half marathons, and full marathons. There is resource information on fat burning, nutrition, motivation, and much more.

Galloway Training Programs
This book has the information you need to train for the classic event: the marathon. It also has schedules for the half marathon and 10-mile race. New in 2007, this has the latest on walk breaks, long runs, practical nutrition, mental marathon toughness, and much more.

Nutrition for Runners
With Nancy Clark (RD)
Using material from renowned nutritionist Nancy Clark, Jeff Galloway gives the reader tips on what to eat, when to eat, how much to eat, and how to combine all that with your training schedule while still retaining the chance to enjoy other aspects of life.

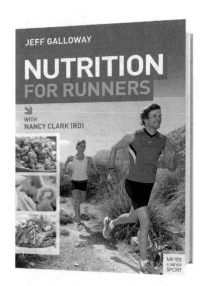

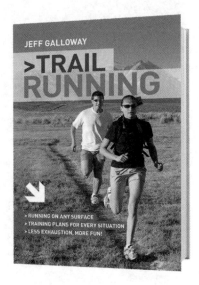

Trail Running
Jeff Galloway teaches you to start trail running the right way with his unique way of guaranteeing an injury free running style. The book covers training plans for beginners and advanced runners as well as a wide range of trail running equipment, especially the whole range of trail running shoes.

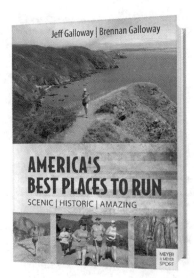

America's Best Places to Run
By Jeff and Brennan Galloway
This book enhances the running experience by offering access to very special running routes. It gives a preview of the scenery with directions to the start and special instructions to enjoy the area. The book also includes tips on training for trail running, dealing with elevation, running uphill and downhill, terrain issues, and endurance.

Running: A Year-Round Plan

This is my most comprehensive training book. It has all of the elements scheduled, leading to goal races of 5K, 10K, half marathon, and marathon within 52 weeks. It weaves the training for several races at one time. You can choose plan A (to finish), plan B (to run a bit better than you are currently running), or plan C (to maximize performance). All of the training elements are scheduled, every day of the year.

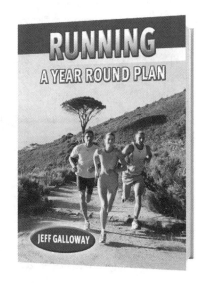

Boston Marathon:
How to Qualify

Galloway's successful training schedules include all of the elements needed to qualify based upon Boston Marathon standards. Galloway's magic mile gives a reality check on progress and sets realistic pacing goals for long runs and the race itself.

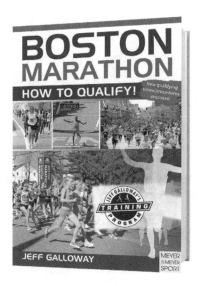

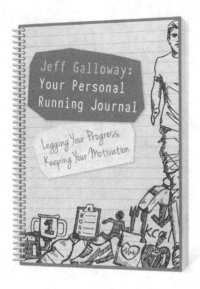

Jeff Galloway's Training Journal

This is an upgraded version of my original training journal (see picture). You'll have one year of log entries with instructions on how to set up training for various goals, analyze data, track performance, etc. This journal can allow you to organize, stay focused on your goal, and evaluate your training. There is also space for recording the unexpected thoughts and experiences that make so many runs come alive again as we read them.

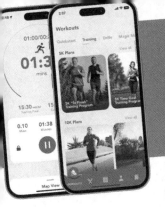

JEFF GALLOWAY

RUN WALK RUN

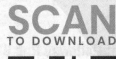

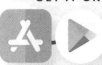
OUR BEST
FEATURES

Magic Mile Test

No need to guess how fast to run when Jeff's Magic Mile helps you dial in the perfect pace for you.

Custom Plans

Programs for any event and fitness level.

Meal Plan

Healthy meals to power your training.

Expert Advice

Daily guidance every step of the way to the finish line.

Complete Control

Customize your workout on the fly to match your needs.

Drills for Skills

Improve your running strength, form and speed.

Track

Track your workouts to see your progress.

Running schools and retreats

I conduct motivating running schools and retreats. These feature individualized information and form evaluation, and comprehensively cover running, nutrition, and fat burning.

Jeff Galloway Run Walk Run app

This is the perfect app for scheduling your run-walk intervals. With the app, you can do a Magic Mile test, customize your own training plans, receive expert advice, use drills to improve your running, follow meal plans, and track your progress. The app is available from the app store, my website *www.jeffgalloway.com*, or you can even scan the QR code on the previous page.

Vitamins

I now believe that most runners need a good vitamin to help the immune system and resist infection. There is some evidence that getting the proper vitamin mix can speed recovery. The vitamin line I use is called Cooper Complete, created by Dr. Kenneth Cooper. In the process of producing the best body of research on exercise and long-term health I've seen anywhere, he has found that certain vitamins help in many ways.

Buffered salt tablets

The most common reason for muscle cramping is not inserting walk breaks early and often enough in long runs and races. But if your muscles continue to cramp on long or hard runs at very short Run Walk Run intervals, buffered salt tablets can probably help. The buffered sodium and potassium tablets get into the system more quickly. Be sure to ask your doctor if this product is okay for you, particularly if you have high blood pressure. If you are taking a statin drug for cholesterol and are cramping, it is doubtful that this will help. Ask your doctor about adjusting the medication before long runs.

Using smartwatches to monitor heart rate

Left-brain runners who are motivated by technical items and data tracking tell me that they are more motivated when using a heart monitor. Right-brain runners who love the intuitive feel of running find that the post-workout number crunching is often too intense, jolting them out of their transcendental state of running. After talking with hundreds of both types of runners, I came to the conclusion that there are benefits to using a heart monitor, especially for runners who are doing speed training.

Once you determine your maximum heart rate, a good heart monitor can help you manage your effort level. This will give you more control over the amount of effort you are spending in a workout, so that you can reduce overwork and recovery time. As they push into the exertion zone needed on a hard workout, left-brain runners will gain a reasonably accurate reading on how much effort to spend or how much they need to back off to avoid a long recovery. Many type-A runners have to be told to back off before they injure themselves. I've heard from countless numbers of these runners who feel that the monitors pay for themselves by telling them exactly how slow to run on easy days and how long to rest between speed repetitions during workouts. Right-brain runners admit that they enjoy getting verification on the intuitive evaluation of effort levels. The bottom line is that monitors can tell you to go slow enough to recover, how long to rest during a speed session, and what your red zone is during a hard speed workout.

All devices have their technical difficulties. Heart monitors can be influenced by local electronic transmissions, and can have mechanical issues. Cellphone towers and even garage door openers can interfere with a monitor on occasion. This is usually an incidental issue, but keep in mind that if you have an abnormal reading—either high or low—it may be a technical abnormality.

Be sure to read the instruction manual thoroughly, particularly the section about how to attach the device to your body for the most accurate reading. If not attached securely, you will miss some beats. This means that you are actually working a lot harder than you think you are.

I suggest that you keep monitoring how you feel at each 5% percentage increase toward your maximum heart rate. Over time, you will get better at the intuitive feel, for example, of an 85% effort when you should be at 80%.

Get tested to determine your maximum heart rate

If you are going to use a heart monitor, you should be tested to find your maximum heart rate. Some doctors—especially cardiologists—will do this for you. Other testing facilities include human performance labs at universities, and some health clubs and YMCAs. It is best to have the test supervised by someone who is trained in cardiovascular issues. Be sure to say that you only need a maximum heart rate test, not a maximum oxygen uptake test. Once you have run for a couple of months with the monitor, you will have a clear idea what your maximum heart rate is from looking at your heart rate during a series of hard runs. Even on the hard speed workouts you can usually sense whether you could have worked yourself harder. But until you have more runs that push you to the limits, assume that your current top heart rate is within a beat or two of your current maximum that has been previously recorded.

Use the percentage of maximum heart rate as your standard

In general you don't want to get above 90% of your maximum heart rate during workouts. At the end of a long training program, this may happen for a short period during a speed workout, but your goal is to keep the percentage between 70% and 80% during the first half of the speed workout or longer run, and minimize the upward drift at the end of the workout.

Computing maximum heart rate percentage

For example, if your maximum heart rate is 200, then:

- 90% is 180

- 80% is 160

- 70% is 140

- 65% is 130

Maximum heart rate for easy days
When in doubt, run slower. One of the major reasons for fatigue, aches and pains, and burnout is not running slowly enough on the recovery and fun days. Most commonly, the rate will increase at the end of a run. If this happens, slow down and take more walk breaks to keep it below 65%.

Maximum heart rate between speed repetitions
To reduce the lingering fatigue that may continue for days after a hard workout, extend the rest interval walk until the heart rate goes down to this 65% level or lower. At the end of the workout, if the heart rate does not drop below this level for 5 minutes, you should do your warm-down and call it a day, even if you have a few repetitions to go.

Maximum heart rate during speed work
Run more smoothly on speed repetitions so that your heart rate stays below 80% during speed work. If you really work on running form improvements, you can minimize the heart rate increase by running more efficiently: keeping feet low to the ground, using a light touch, maintaining quick but efficient turnover of the feet. For more info on this, see chapter 11, or *Galloway's Book on Running, Second Edition*.

Morning pulse

If the chest strap doesn't interfere with your sleep, you can get a very accurate reading on your resting pulse in the morning. This will allow you to monitor overtraining. Record the low figures each night. Once you establish a baseline, you should take an easy day when the rate rises 5-9% above this. When it reaches 10% or above, you should take an extra day off. Even if the heart rate increase is due to an infection, you should not run unless cleared by your doctor.

Two-minute rule for long runs

Use the two-minute rule for the pace of long runs, not heart rate. Even when running at 65% of maximum heart rate, many runners will be running a lot faster than they should at the beginning of long runs. Read the guidelines in this book for pacing the long runs, and don't be bashful about running slower. At the end of long runs, remember to back off when your heart rate exceeds 70% of the maximum heart rate. There will be some upward drift of heart rate due to fatigue at the end of long runs. Keep slowing down if this happens, so that you stay around 70% or lower of your maximum heart rate, even during the last few miles.

GPS and other distance-pace calculators

There are two types of devices for measuring distance, and both are usually very accurate: GPS and accelerometer technology. While some devices are more accurate than others, most will tell you almost exactly how far you have run. This provides the best pacing feedback I know of—except for running on a track—so that you don't start your runs too fast, etc.

Using more accurate products gives you freedom. You can do your long runs without having to measure the course or being forced to run on a repeated—but measured—loop. Instead of going to a track to do speed sessions, you can very quickly measure your segments on roads, trails, or residential streets with GPS devices. If your goal race is on the track, I recommend that at least half of your speed sessions be run on the track. This relates to the principle of training called *specificity*.

The GPS devices track your movements by the use of navigational satellites. In general, the more satellites, the more accurate the measurement. There are shadows—areas of buildings, forests, or mountains—in many areas where the signal cannot be acquired for (usually) short distances. You can see how accurate they are by running around a standard track. If you run in the middle of the first lane (not right next to the inside) you will be running about .25 mile.

The accelerometer products require a very easy calibration and have been shown to be very accurate. I've found it best to use a variety of paces and a walk break or two on the calibration in order to simulate what you will be doing when you run.

Most smartwatches and smartphones come equip with GPS and can monitor heart rate. Check in with fellow runners to see what apps they prefer to use to monitor heart rate.

The Galloway Run Walk Run App

• Timers take the guesswork out of Run Walk Run. I have created my very own Run Walk Run app which is perfect for tracking your running and walking intervals.

• Those who have trouble taking the walk breaks early in the runs find that they become like one of Pavlov's dogs as they reprogram the subconscious brain. You don't have to stress over walk breaks when you're using the app.

• You can easily adjust your Run Walk Run strategy using the tips provided in the app.

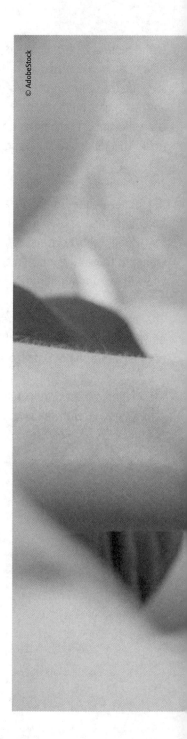

© AdobeStock

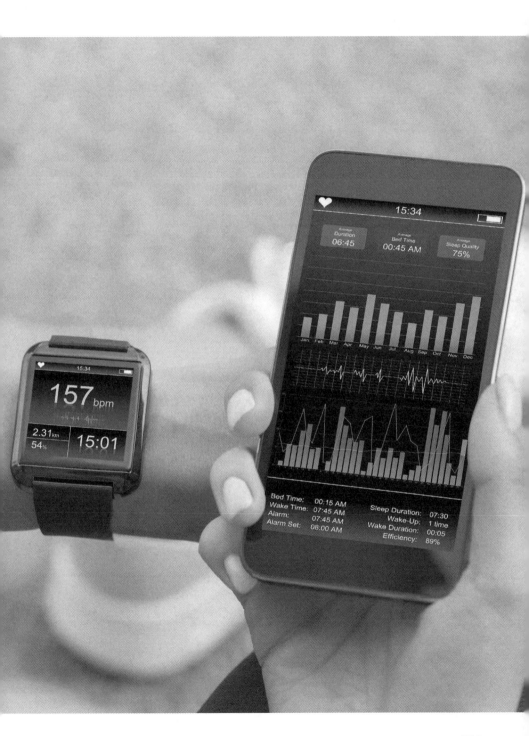

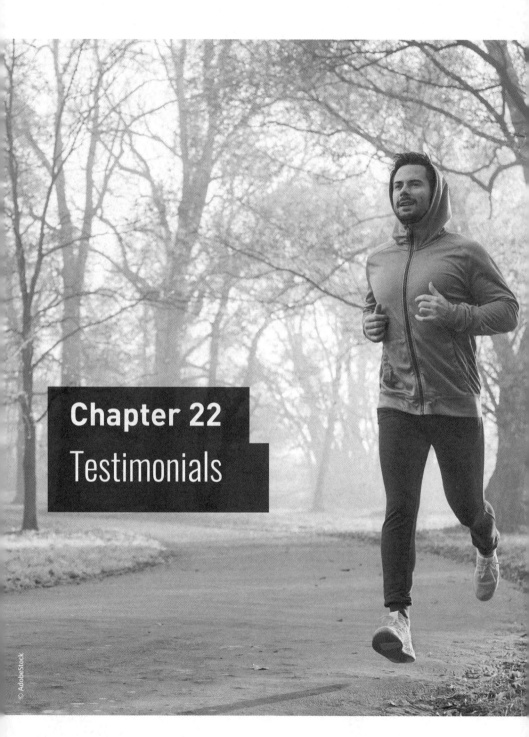

Chapter 22
Testimonials

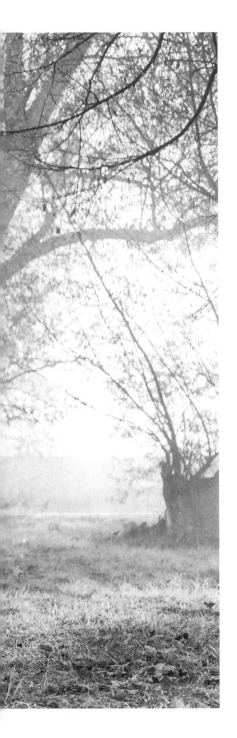

Thousands of runners tell me every year that they started running only because they discovered my Run Walk Run method. Until then, most thought that you had to run continuously in order to be considered a runner and they originally tried to do this. When they became winded, exhausted, sore, or nauseous they assumed that their bodies weren't designed for running.

Everything changed when they started inserting walk breaks after a few minutes (or a few seconds) into the run; huffing and puffing stopped, pain went away, and muscles were strong to the finish. Replacing the negatives was the glow of accomplishment, a better attitude, and vitality that enhanced their run and their life. YOU CAN TOO!

I doubt that you will find any training component that will help you in more ways than my Run Walk Run method. I continue to be amazed, every week, at the reports of how strategic walk breaks help runners enjoy every run—even those which started to be difficult. When placed appropriately for the individual, walk breaks erase debilitating tiredness, reduce stress, improve motivation, increase running enjoyment and speed of recovery, and allow the runner to finish with strength.

Some of the stories below deal with the shift in mental activity when you have a strategy of Run Walk Run or change it. When we start any run, the subconscious brain uses existing patterns of motion learned in childhood, on a sports team, etc., when the current physical capabilities are not what they were back then. Stress builds up quickly and the subconscious brain will trigger the release of negative attitude hormones.

By focusing on the Run Walk Run method and monitoring the amount of running and walking, you shift mental action out of the subconscious brain and into your frontal lobe, the strategy center. This allows you to control your pace and your comfort zone. Conscious activity in the frontal lobe overrides the subconscious reflex brain and puts you in control of your workout and your life.

Many of the folks below appreciate the control. Others are struck by the amazing feeling of strength to the end with quick recovery. By having a strategy, monitoring your breathing, and making adjustments, you can stay mentally focused. There is no need to be totally exhausted at the end of any long run.

One of the first success stories is my own: In 1980, I ran my best marathon time, 2:16, in the Houston Tenneco Marathon. I took walk breaks every 2 miles from the beginning and improved my PR by 2 minutes!

"I don't have to run a marathon...only one minute at a time."

Elaine W.

Elaine used to have to walk the last 2-3 miles of every marathon. By running a minute and walking a minute she focused on each run segment to the finish line. She explained how the accomplishment gave meaning to the long journey of training and empowered her to make several significant changes in other areas of life.

- -

"I had trouble running around the block when I was just running without walk breaks. I just ran a half marathon on Saturday and a marathon today because of your method."

John B.

John assumed his running days were over because he couldn't run continuously—even around his suburban block of less than half a mile. When his sister signed up for the Walt Disney World Goofy Challenge, he couldn't understand it. In high school, Sis couldn't make it through gym class. She explained to John how you can melt the fatigue and stress of any distance by running a short segment and then walking to erase the running fatigue. Sis started with 20 seconds running and 40 seconds walking which worked for John also. He used this to get through all of the training, and the two events on race weekend—back to back.

- -

"I promised my kids that we would go to all of the Disney parks after I ran my race, the Disney Princess Half Marathon. Here I am, having fun. I have at least as much energy as they do."

Terri S .

Terri is one of the growing number of moms who have found that kids will put up with months of training, being late for breakfast on long run mornings, etc. if they get to go to Disney World. She discovered that Run Walk Run never compromised her family or other activities even after the really long training runs. After the Disney Princess Half Marathon she went all over Disney World and enjoyed being with the kids.

-- --

"I surprised myself today—I qualified for Boston after ten years of trying. My big breakthrough with your method was understanding that I could change the ratio and feel better right away. I shifted from R4min/W1min to R2min/W30sec, and picked up speed."

Bob C.

Running continuously during a segment that is too long for you on that day will result in extreme fatigue, slowdown, and physical exhaustion. There is no ratio that is set in stone. Not only did Bob reduce his fatigue by cutting running and walking segments in half, he felt the empowerment of taking control over his race strategy with more frequent walks before he was exhausted and eliminated a slowdown at the end.

-- --

"Call me what you will but I like to be in control of how I feel. Your method gives me permission to adjust as I go to feel good from start to finish."

Susan M.

The human psyche wants to be in control. Probably the best benefit of Run Walk Run is that you are in command of how you feel during and after a run. You can enjoy the endorphins that are produced by the run while avoiding the negatives of overexertion. Each time you walk you exercise your power during that moment—and can stay in control to the end of the run and throughout the rest of the day.

- -

"I run to deal with stress. When running without walk breaks, I increased stress. My walk breaks bring joy while releasing the tension from the stress of the day."

Paul S.

Walk breaks dissolve two types of stress: physical and psychological. Stress to the muscles, tendons, joints, and nerves can be managed with the appropriate Run Walk Run strategy for the day. Lowering the physical stress will lower the psychological stress. This means that you can reduce the negative attitude hormones and allow the positive endorphins to lock into receptors and send messages of well-being.

- -

"I ran in college for fitness but couldn't run very far and I never walked. It hurt after a while so I quit for 15 years. My sister told me about your technique and the short segments of running brought me back to the best part of my college running—being in the moment. Each run is an opportunity to experience the wonderful gift of physical exertion. Each walk allows me to reflect on this."

Barbara C

From breast cancer and open heart surgery to the marathon!

When 4-year breast cancer survivor Nancy P. started training with the Galloway Program in Jacksonville, FL, for the Marathon to Finish Breast Cancer, she inspired her 80-year-old father to experiment with various walk breaks. Nancy was sailing along using R1min/W1min while her father, a survivor of open-heart surgery, tried various ratios on his own. Unfortunately the R1min/W1min was too much for Nancy, and she incurred a stress fracture on the 14-mile run. After a 6-week healing break from running, she conferred with me about the possibility of resuming her goal after the setback. She didn't like what I told her:

"His plan sounded CRAZY! He wanted me to walk the first 10 miles of my next 16-mile long run and then do R15sec/W45sec for the last 6. I couldn't believe it! Going from the R1min/W1min and not being particularly fast and now shifting to R15sec/W45sec, I wondered how in the world was going to work.

"I showed the plan to my dad and after some discussion we reminded ourselves that Jeff literally wrote the book on the Run Walk Run method so he must know what he's doing. We decided to give it a try. Dad and I went out with the Galloway group on a Saturday morning. We positioned ourselves right behind the R1min/W1min marathon group and right in front of the R1min/W1:30min marathon group. To our surprise, we stayed right between them the whole way. This new method hadn't changed my pace at all. Wow!"

So Dad got inspired! Nancy was reenergized and her dad was a bit too inspired and tried to maintain a stride that was too long, pulling a muscle—but he was back after his healing vacation, and continued to train. Various muscle issues caused him to think that the half marathon was a better choice for him, even if he didn't like it.

But during the last few days before the race, they had a strategy session, did the math on per mile pace, and he believed he could finish the marathon. Using R15sec/W45sec, father and daughter pulled one another along to the finish together.

**"I owe my recovery to you and your Run Walk Run process!
I am living proof of it!"**

Jim B.

In spite of over 20 years of running, Jim was told by his doctor in 2005 that he had serious coronary heart disease and needed immediate open-heart surgery to save his life. As he began his return to exercise, he attended one of my running schools and saw the Run Walk Run method as the best way to return to running. He has continued to benefit and has made a strong comeback: three marathons and over a dozen half marathons with lots of other races.

Amazingly strong at the finish—could run the next day

"I was broken down, undertrained, and mentally down, but wanted to finish the Walt Disney World Marathon. Because my pride had been damaged, I was ready to use Run Walk Run for the first time and talked to you at the expo. I was surprised that you only wanted me to run for two minutes, then walk for a minute. I struggled with this but realized that I would probably not finish if I did it my way.

Everything you said was 100% right on. I was so strong at the finish it amazed me. The last two miles I ran in under 8:00 pace.

I felt the very best that I have ever felt after a full marathon. I was recovered and ready to run the following morning (but didn't). No question, your system works and I have just become one of your biggest supporters."

Robert P.

A love/love relationship with running because of Run Walk Run

"I heard you speak at the Big Sur expo in 2008 and decided to try the Run Walk Run thing for the race the next day. Coming from Ohio, my hill training wasn't up to par and I knew the walk breaks were going to help me endure the rugged course and that's exactly what they did. I had a blast at the race and felt awesome, meanwhile my husband had to get fluids in the med tent. He did not take walk breaks.

Needless to say I stuck with the method and have watched my love-hate relationship with running turn into a love-love relationship. I've PR'd in my last two races and simply feel great! Life with less fatigue is wonderful. I've also started coaching a 5K team in town and we teach them to run by alternating between running and walking.

Just wanted to say thanks and share my story. I wouldn't be the runner I am today without that chance meeting and hearing you speak at Big Sur a few years ago. That drop in the water is still rippling."

Hannah

No more hip pain!

"Just wanted to give you an update on your suggestions from the Nashville running school. If you will remember, my hip was hurting after the long runs and you suggested I use R15sec/W45sec for the next long run. Well, JoAnne and I tried it in our long run and it was a great warm-up but after about a mile we could hardly stand to stop at the 15 seconds so we changed it to R20sec/W40sec and truly that is the happy pace for us. We end up gliding at the end of the 20 seconds to transition into the walk more easily. It was fantastic! We had never had such an enjoyable run. We did the R20sec/W40sec in the half marathon in B'ham this last weekend and it was awesome! My hip did not hurt at all at the end and we finished in 2:50:49 which was perfectly on our 13-minute pace with a hill that was about 2 miles long. We are so psyched to do it again. Wow, thanks for the great advice."

Robin

- -

"Your training programs have gotten me to where I am today. I couldn't run a quarter of a mile, now I'm a Boston Qualifier."

Jim

- -

"Run Walk Run has revolutionized my running. I can't believe....

1. How great I feel at the end of each walking break when I start running again.

2. How good I feel the rest of the day as well as the next after a long run."

Kevin

Running faster and feeling better with Run Walk Run

"I started running for the first time in my life about a year ago as a way to fight the boredom of the bike, treadmill, and stair stepper at the gym. I gradually increased my distance to 5 miles, running non-stop. A friend recommended your book on running and I read it and it made a lot of sense, so I started right away with the R3min/W1min ratio. From my first run using the Run Walk Run method, my times were faster and I felt better. So I started to increase my distance just for fun to see how far I could go. Once I got over 7-8 miles, I bought your half marathon book and started to train for a half marathon in September. And my mileage just kept increasing while I was still feeling good, so I bought your marathon book and trained for a full marathon in November and ran it only 6 months after starting to run for the first time in my life! I'm a big believer in the Run Walk Run method for making running enjoyable and staying injury-free!!! I also admit to following all your advice for the to-finish marathon and that really helped. I'm so glad I just focused on finishing and making it fun. Now I want to do it again (and maybe even improve on my time)!"

Allison R

No asthma attacks!

"Recently, I was hit with pneumonia and was out of running for a month only to find that when I started running again, my old methods left me with an asthma attack. I realized I needed to look into other methods of training. I discovered your podcasts and LOVE them! The first time I used the 30 seconds run/ 30 seconds walk, I was able to go the distance without fatigue and no asthma attacks!"

D. C.

Amazing results when undertrained

"Six weeks before the marathon I became injured. I trained very little during the last 6 weeks but did a 12 mile non-stop run one week before. At the expo, you told me to run a minute/walk a minute. I had never tried Run Walk Run so I gave it a try and was able to increase the running during the race to 2 minutes.

I did this up to mile 20 and ran the rest of the way. I felt great the whole race and strong at the end running mile 25 at an 8:20 pace. You said you wanted me to have a good race, and I DID! I remain injury free and the course was spectacular. My time was 4:06 with the first half at 2:03—so I ran an even split."

Dean S.

Attitude improvement

"Run Walk Run has given me control over my training, my attitude, and my life. I never expected the changes to my outlook on life. What a pleasant surprise. And the best thing about it is that it is something that will never go away. I'll always know what I've been able to accomplish and that I can do whatever I set my mind to."

B. T.

Family runs together with Run Walk Run

"By using R30sec/W30sec, my husband Bill, my 12-year-old son Reid, and I finished the half marathon 12 minutes faster than expected. It was a big first half marathon for Reid and Bill who started running after a serious brain tumor challenge. Bill said, I used to proudly tell people that my wife is a runner. Now I can proudly tell them that I'm a runner, too. I'm still on that endorphin high!"

A. C.

"We were middle-aged guys who had come to realize that the only way we were going to set a personal best at our age was to do something we'd never done before."

I've never been a strong runner. I joined my high school cross-country team not for love of running, but because of a girl. (She was faster than me, so the strategy didn't really work out.) My relationship with running has always been what you could call complicated; I liked the effect, but not so much the cause. I even stopped running for 10 years or so with the excuse that my knees hurt, or some such thing.

Then about 5 years ago, someone at work said he was going to run the Big Sur Marathon. I said I admired his lunacy, but he said it wasn't that hard. He said he followed the Galloway Method. He explained that he alternated running and walking intervals, and that he was able to go farther than he ever could without stopping. So I went for a run with him—expecting to be thoroughly humiliated by a guy 15 years my junior—and I was hooked. I started a recreational running club at work. When we're having a particularly difficult time on our Sunday long run, we'll just say to each other "What would Jeff do?" or "Remember what Jeff says: Obey your body" or "In Galloway we trust."

Don't get me wrong. We weren't zealots looking for a spiritual guide. We were middle-aged guys who had come to realize that the only way we were going to set a personal best at our age was to do something we'd never done before. And even though I'll never qualify for Boston, running has given me life memories I'll always cherish."

E. B.

Run Walk Run improves running and life

"It wasn't an easy decision for me to embrace your program fully, but it was one of the best decisions I have ever made. Every promise you make in your books and at your clinics about the impact of your method on one's running and one's life is coming true for me. I really can't begin to thank you enough."

A. C.

- -

Forty-five pounds lighter and now a marathoner

"Jeff, your methods and education have changed my life forever. In just one year, I went from 44 years old and ZERO exercise for the past 20 years to 45 lbs. lighter and just ran a 4:41 marathon. Resting heart rate went from 80 BPM down to 52 BPM."

T.K.

- -

Others are inspired to exercise because of Run Walk Run

"Because of my success with your method, my dad (>70) is planning to do a 5k with me, a friend who never ran before is running 20ish miles, my best man in my wedding, who never ran, is doing the Army 10 miler with me (with his 13 year old daughter), a long time friend who was about 350 pounds has started running, has done two 5ks and has started to lose weight, two neighbors and a friend of mine have completed the Marine Corps marathon, and a small group of women from church have started to run as well.

All this has happened using your books and methods and the learning I've received from your coaching. It's really cool."

S. T.

Total change in attitude!

"The last six months following the Run Walk Run program have been amazing. After an unpleasant divorce and two miserable years, I am happy and healthy and training for the marathon was a big part of that."

D. M.

New life after a tragedy

"My son was killed in Iraq 4 years ago and as you would expect I crawled into a dark hole. A year ago another mom who had also lost her son in Iraq convinced me that I should try running. I laughed because I have never run beyond what was mandated in school PE, but she was convincing. I found your program online and decided to give it a try. Our plan was to run the Marine Corps Marathon this year to honor our sons—a very lofty goal—so I registered for the marathon and your local training program.

I had the opportunity to meet you and hear you speak when we kicked off the spring program here in Salt Lake. I reluctantly attended the seminar because I looked about as far from a runner as you can get. I was truly inspired to hear you speak; you answered my questions and not once did I feel like I didn't belong with the group. I bought several of your books on getting started and nutrition; both are well-worn and have been a constant go-to this year. Your directors here in Salt Lake took it from there. Angie Whitworth and Jim Levy were there for me every step of the way. Not once this year did I feel like I could not reach my goal even though it was tough. I followed your program to the letter and never missed a run.

Before your program I was not able to run to the end of my street, but I kept going. I have lost almost 70 lbs. since I met you earlier this year and have run three marathons, including the Marine Corps Marathon I had planned to honor my son. I have five more races planned for the upcoming year and I have truly found a passion for running through your program.

You need to know that while I will forever miss my son, I can see the sunlight again. I am healthy, I am a runner, I am a marathoner, and I have a new passion for life. I owe all of this to you, Angie, Jim, and your program. Thank you, you all will forever have a special place in my heart!"

T. D.

Attitude change and 80 pounds lighter

"My exposure to your Run Walk Run philosophy has truly impacted the person I am today. I no longer dread getting up to run. In fact, I cannot stand to miss it! About a year ago I couldn't even run 20 seconds without stopping. The other morning I was at the track and I was running my 6th 400. I ran it in 2:19!

My weight continues to go down. I weigh less now that I have in about 5 years. If I drop 20 more pounds (my goal) I will have lost 100 pounds since the height of my pregnancy! So I just keep on trucking!!

Thank you again for your guidance, friendship, and inspiration. You have inspired me to be an athlete again and I cannot shake this running bug I caught from YOU."

A.K.

Life change

"I just wanted to let you know that your Run Walk Run method has changed my life. (A little dramatic maybe? No. Not really.)

I started running at 48. I've never been an athlete—in fact, I smoked for 16 years. Sedentary life caused a weight gain in my 30s and 40s. I lost some weight when I was 47, decided that to keep it off I needed to up my exercise, and thought I'd try running.

So without any coaching or knowledge I tried. I couldn't even run to the church—less than 300 meters away! I slowed down and persisted though, as I had an event in honor of a dear friend's daughter who passed away from cancer at 21, and I was GOING to run that 5k for her! I read and trained, and trained some more, and eventually could run 5K without stopping, but not without injury. I ran the 5K and was hooked on running, so two months later attempted a 10K (Can you say overtraining??) and sidelined myself really well with a severe plantar fascia injury. Ugh. It was so bad I could barely walk. I went to physio for 6 weeks and it took another 6 before I was allowed to run for even a minute. It took about 6 months for the injury to heal completely. What did I learn? I was never going to let THAT happen again! (And I learned I was really hooked on running and really, really still wanted to run!)

So I started searching the net for ways to run without injury and guess whose name popped up again and again?? I thought, "This make sense! I can do this, after all, I'm very good at walking!"

I read everything I could find on the net by you. I bought a couple of your books and an interval timer and I was off! (This was about November/December 2011).

I used your method to train over our long cold winter here in eastern Ontario, Canada. I ran and walked in the rain and the snow and I had a good time doing it! (Every run I find something pretty, fun, and inspiring to enjoy). I had a goal in mind and I have reached it. Last weekend I ran the Ottawa Half Marathon in 2:38! I ran according to what my body was telling me and I came in strong and happy! I had lots of energy after the race (once I'd cooled down) and went on to enjoy my day with my family and friends.

Well, you know the sense of pride I feel at setting and then achieving such an unfathomable (just a few years ago) goal, and I'm still flying high. I think a marathon may even be in my distant future but I'll revisit that another day. I certainly can see a few more half marathons in my life to help me maintain my fitness. (I love a goal to work to.) And I might even do that negative split when I run a half in the fall when the weather is a little better for runners.

I just wanted to say thanks, you've made such a difference in my life and in the lives of many, many others."

K. R.

Run Walk Run makes it possible to enjoy accomplishment

"I met you at the Nashville Fleet Feet a few months ago. I told you then that I was a newbie, inspired by your Run Walk Run method to continue in this sport. I had to complete your 5K training program three times before I felt I could attempt a race, but my wife and I did a 5K race in Knoxville, then the Expedition Everest 5K Challenge in Walt Disney World, and now we're both completely hooked. I'm 51 years old, but I intend to run every Disney race—that's my bucket list.

I started running simply to drop a few pounds and get my blood pressure under control. All that was achieved in the first few months. And by then, I was addicted! If I miss a run now, I feel deeply disappointed in myself. I constantly bore non-runners with all my running talk. My proudest possession is my Forerunner. And I've read all your books at least four times. I have tons of mental tricks to get myself through the tough miles, thanks to your suggestions and your book *Mental Training for Runners*. (My autographed copy is completely dog-earred.) The trick that works best for me: I started track in middle school because I was intrigued by the Steve Prefontaine articles in Sports Illustrated back then, so I'm fond of saying "Pre Lives" out loud. It's always good for a few more run segments, even if other people look at me like I'm insane. Heck, I know I'll get plenty of those looks anyway! And I often pretend that you're running right beside me, making sure I don't run the run segments too fast. Especially in those first few miles. That truly works for me. If the teacher is right beside the pupil, the pupil is far more attentive and obedient, right?

I just wanted to take a few minutes to thank you for your advice, enthusiasm, and encouragement. I'm thoroughly hooked on running now. HEALTHY running, the Galloway Way. All I want is to someday be able to keep up a 10-minute pace. And if that day never comes, I can content myself with my 12:30 pace."

T.M.

Strong to the finish

"I decided to try your Run Walk Run method in a race (heretofore I couldn't bring myself to walk in the early miles), and it really worked wonders. The race was a 20-miler, and I used it as a prep for this fall's Twin Cities Marathon (I hope at some point you can come back to the Twin Cities). At the half marathon point I noticed my time was a bit better than the two previous half marathons I had run just weeks earlier. The biggest improvements were that I felt relatively strong at the finish instead of feeling like I was starting to fall apart, and the diminished muscle soreness (no ibuprofen afterward....that's a first!) really has me hooked! Even though it is hard to take breaks in the early miles, I know it's really worth it. As I get older, I have much more confidence that your method will help me run stronger and longer. I deeply appreciate all of the credence you have brought to the Run Walk Run method as it's helped make the sport of running much more accessible and enjoyable!"

S. F.

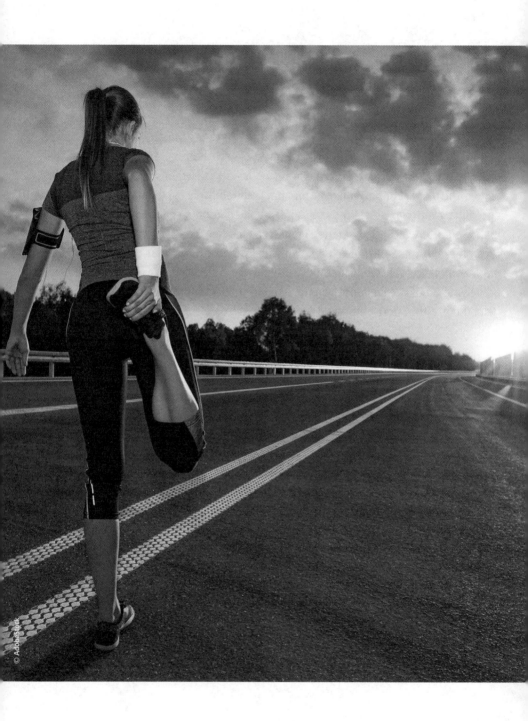

© AdobeStock

Run Walk Run: Focus on a different kind of success

"I am 61 years old and for about 20 years was an avid (and successful runner—qualifying for Boston Marathon in a time of 3:43). Sometime in my later 40s, I slacked off my running due to heavy workload and Atlanta commute times and within another couple years was having knee, hip, and back pain whenever I tried to run with any regularity. I had almost given up on running when I heard you speak at the CDC Lifestyle Fitness Center in the spring of 2010. After you spoke, I explained to you in an aside that I used to be a fast runner (with a 7-min/mile pace) and asked how should I go about regaining that speed now that I was almost 60. I will never forget your response—"You don't. Don't try. You will get a career-ending injury."

That was probably the single best piece of running advice I ever received! After that, I bought your *Running Until You're 100* and started using the Run Walk Run method. I love it! It gets me out the door even when I am not sure I feel like running. I have completed a number of 5Ks and one 15K in the past couple of years and had fun doing it.

This year I set a goal to do three successively longer triathlons (haven't done longer than a sprint triathlon in 17 years and had never done a half ironman before). I registered for the Augusta 70.3 Half Ironman and successfully completed the 1.2-mile swim, 56-mile bike and 13.1-mile run in 6:25:50. I won third place in my age group (3 out of 6). For a slower swimmer, this was phenomenal!

When I got off the bike, my right quad immediately cramped up into a huge ball, but I didn't panic. I changed into running shoes and, knowing I had adequate electrolytes, fluids, and glucose on board and months of Galloway training behind me, I confidently began the half marathon. I was only able to jog 20 seconds at a time for the first few minutes, but gradually felt better and ended up using my usual R3-5min/W45sec and finished the run in 2:20 with a 10:43 per mile pace. And I had fun along the way!

Just wanted to say thanks for helping me regain my motivation and a totally different perspective on succeeding at running. This is much more fun without the race day jitters!"

C. H.

Comeback after open-heart surgery

"I successfully used your Run Walk Run timer to complete the Walla Walla, WA, Marathon on October 14. I had open-heart surgery last year to remove a blood clot from my pulmonary artery. The damage to my left lung was severe, so breathing during times of exertion is difficult. I was able to use the timer during training to determine my best running to recovery ratio. I use R1:12min/W2min and I am proud to say my time was 6:29:18."

R.S.

Five quality marathons in one year without hitting the wall

Joe Ely recently sent me a report of his experiments with various strategies using Run Walk Run since 2007. In 2012 he tested the system, running 5 marathons. Here's how it went:

First was the Carmel Marathon on April 21, 2012 in suburban Indianapolis. Joe used R6min/W1min through mile 24.5, then ran it in. This yielded an official time of 4:33:25—at the time his second best marathon of this running era, plus a 3-second negative split.

Marathon 2 was the Bayshore Marathon in Traverse City, MI. Since he was running a trail marathon two weeks later, he took a then-radical plan to shift his pace. His plan was to use R3min/W1min through mile 10, then R4min/W1min to the finish. As it played out, he felt so good, he ran the last 2.2 miles and finished in 4:40:16, with almost 4-minute negative split. This was his second race in a row with no wall, feeling marvelous at the end.

Joe felt that his slow, conservative start did nothing to diminish his overall time and actually served as a governor to hold him back in the face of the adrenaline of a big race in a beautiful setting. This confirms much of what I have been saying for years. Interestingly, when he shifted to R4min/W1min, he didn't really budge his overall average mile pace very much.

Marathon 3 was the Wineglass Marathon in Corning, NY. Because his next marathon was only 7 days later, Joe ran R3min/W1min through mile 16, shifted to R4min/W1min, and then ran the last 3 miles non-stop with a finish time of 4:38:55 and another negative split. He said he felt "awesome at the end...still no wall, still no cramps, a truly fun marathon."

Marathon 4 was a big one, the Chicago Marathon. Because he had never run marathons one week apart he used R3min/W1min through mile 20, shifted to R4min/W1min, and realized his finish vision for that race: to run, continuously, the final 3+ miles down Michigan Avenue for a 4:48:28 and an 8-minute negative split). Because of the weaving in this crowded race, Joe probably ran a mile farther, and had a 6-minute port-a-potty stop, so his actual 26.2-mile time was comparable to his finish the week before. The best part is that he "felt terrific at the end and truly enjoyed this world-class event."

Marathon 5 of the year's journey was the Chicamauga Battlefield Marathon. He ran with two friends who were walking 30 seconds every mile but realized at about 4.5 miles that this wasn't working and dropped back to R3min/W1min through mile 13. At that point he shifted to R4min/W1min through mile 24 and ran to the finish. The lack of adequate walk breaks in the beginning resulted in foot and calf cramps at the end, but he recorded his second fastest marathon of his mature era, 4:27:32. Joe says that's "not bad for a 59-year-old guy!"

Index

5K Program 62

B
Beginners 47, 59
Brain Programming 21, 30

D
Downhill Running 52
Drills Acceleration Glider 77
Drills Cadence 75

E
Endorphines 27, 31
Energy Consumption 13

F
First Time Racers 42

G
Gadgets and apps 55, 138

H
Half Marathon 43
Heart Rate 155
Heart Monitors 156
Hills 95

I
Injuries 33, 84
Interval Training 25

L

Leap of Faith 43
Long Run 98

M

Magic Mile 37
Mental Benefits 25, 29
Mental Performance 121
Micro Tears 35
Motivation 121
Muscle Fatigue 25

O

Orthopedic Stress 13

P

Pace Per Mile 63
Pain Reduction 82
Performance Prediction 40
Pulse 158

R

Race Rehearsal 113
Recovery 26, 89, 135
Run Walk Run Intervals 135
Run Walk Run Method 15
Run Walk Run Strategies 48
Runners, Heavy 101
Runners, Older 102
Running Faster 109, 117
Running Goals 60
Running Injury Free 87
Running Posture 68
Running Segments 122

S

Subconscious 21

T

Temperature Body 27, 94
Temperature 47, 94
Training Schedule, 5K 65
Training Schedule, Catch Up 99

U

Uphill Running 51

W

Walk Breaks 16, 30, 67
Walk Faster 73
Walking 15, 71, 105
Walking Form 71
Warm-up 64
Weak Links 13, 26, 33

Credits

Cover design:	Anja Elsen
Interior design and layout:	Anja Elsen
Cover photo:	© AdobeStock
Interior photos:	© AdobeStock
Copy Editor:	Anne Rumery